Happiness—Concept, Measurement and Promotion

Yew-Kwang Ng

Happiness—Concept, Measurement and Promotion

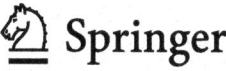 Springer

Yew-Kwang Ng
School of Economics
Fudan University
Shanghai, China

Economics
Monash University
Melbourne, Australia

ISBN 978-981-33-4971-1   ISBN 978-981-33-4972-8 (eBook)
https://doi.org/10.1007/978-981-33-4972-8

© The Editor(s) (if applicable) and The Author(s) 2022. This book is an open access publication.
Open Access This book is licensed under the terms of the Creative Commons Attribution 4.0 International License (http://creativecommons.org/licenses/by/4.0/), which permits use, sharing, adaptation, distribution and reproduction in any medium or format, as long as you give appropriate credit to the original author(s) and the source, provide a link to the Creative Commons license and indicate if changes were made.
The images or other third party material in this book are included in the book's Creative Commons license, unless indicated otherwise in a credit line to the material. If material is not included in the book's Creative Commons license and your intended use is not permitted by statutory regulation or exceeds the permitted use, you will need to obtain permission directly from the copyright holder.
The use of general descriptive names, registered names, trademarks, service marks, etc. in this publication does not imply, even in the absence of a specific statement, that such names are exempt from the relevant protective laws and regulations and therefore free for general use.
The publisher, the authors and the editors are safe to assume that the advice and information in this book are believed to be true and accurate at the date of publication. Neither the publisher nor the authors or the editors give a warranty, expressed or implied, with respect to the material contained herein or for any errors or omissions that may have been made. The publisher remains neutral with regard to jurisdictional claims in published maps and institutional affiliations.

This Springer imprint is published by the registered company Springer Nature Singapore Pte Ltd.
The registered company address is: 152 Beach Road, #21-01/04 Gateway East, Singapore 189721, Singapore

Preface

While interests in issues pertaining to happiness have been long-standing, we have witnessed recently an increasing focus by both scholars and members of the general public. 'Subjective well-being (SWB) is an extremely active area of research with about 170,000 articles and books published on the topic in the past 15 years' (Diener et al. 2018, Abstract). Not only psychologists (e.g. Kahneman et al. 1999, Diener et al. 2010, 2018) and sociologists (e.g. Veenhoven 1984, 1993, 2010, 2017), but also economists have made substantial investigations.[1] After about 2–3 decades of gestation since the first publication on happiness issues by an economist (Easterlin 1974), contributions from economists has mushroomed over the last two decades or so.[2] I published a paper (Ng 1978) four years after Easterlin and continue to maintain interest until now. In this book, I hope to show how an individual and a society/country may increase happiness. Despite the fact that happiness has a genetic element (Lykken & Tellegen 1996, Lyubomirsky & Layous 2013, Minkov & Bond 2017), it can be increased (Lyubomirsky 2005, Carrillo et al. 2020);[3] one may even learn or be trained to be happier (e.g. Loveday et al. 2018, Rowland & Curry 2018, Ruch et al. 2018, Liu et al. 2020). At least for myself, my happiness has increased by many times since its low (but still positive) during my early thirties. I hope that many readers may learn from this book to achieve the same or even larger successes. My advice is not just based on my personal experience, but also on the research findings of many researchers from whom I have learned enormously. I believe that this book is useful not only for an individual wishing to increase happiness, or for a government willing to do good for the people, but also for a happiness researcher and an economist if she wants her economics to contribute to social welfare. (On the

---

[1] For a bibliometric analysis of the economics of happiness, see Dominko & Verbič (2019), which shows, among others, a big surge after the global financial crisis in 2008.

[2] Including: Frey & Stutzer (2002), Blanchflower & Oswald (2004), Layard (2006), Clark (2010), Helliwell (2010, 2018), Oswald & Wu (2010), Benjamin et al. (2012, 2014), Graham (2012), 2017), Blanchflower et al. (2013), Clark & Senik (2014), Aghion et al (2016), Cheng et al. (2017), Clark et al. (2018), Glover & Helliwell (2019).

[3] However, see Brown & Rohrer (2020) for a critical comment on Lyubomirsky (2005).

other hand, the concern for the danger of a paternalistic government should also be kept in mind; see, e.g. Frey 2018).

Highlights of the book include:

- A simple, intuitive definition of happiness without the confusion of the objective and/or eudaimonic complications.
- Clarifications on some mistaken views on happiness, such as: happiness is relative, differs between individuals, cannot be measured in a single dimension and cannot be compared interpersonally.
- A sophisticated method to measure happiness (including by survey questionnaire) that is more reliable and interpersonally comparable is proposed.
- The philosophical position that happiness is ultimately speaking the only thing of intrinsic value is strongly defended. This does not preclude important instrumental values of happiness, including for health, success in career and family, productivity or work performance (DiMaria et al. 2020, Luna-Arocas & Danvila-del-Valle 2020) and even in pro-environmental behaviour (e.g. Diener & Tay 2017, Schmitt et al. 2017, Frey 2018, Wang & Kang 2018).
- An environmentally responsible happy nation index (ERHNI): A national success indicator other than GDP.
- An evolutionary ultimate explanation for the delay in sleep-wake cycles of teenagers, explaining the decline in happiness starting at around 12 years old and the trough in happiness levels at middle ages, as well as an obvious way to solve the problems by delaying the start hours of high schools.
- The East-Asian happiness gap.
- Twelve factors: attitude, balance, confidence, dignity, engagement, family/friends, gratitude, health, ideal, joy, kindness, love, crucial for individual happiness.
- Important public policy considerations are discussed, taking into account recent contributions in economics, environmental sciences and happiness studies.
- Arguments very different from, if not opposite to the traditional economist wisdom like 'big society, small government', are advanced.
- A case for brain stimulation for pleasure is made.
- A case for reducing animal suffering.

Shanghai, China   Yew-Kwang Ng

References

AGHION, Philippe, AKCIGIT, Ufuk, DEATON, Angus & ROULET, Alexandra. (2016). Creative destruction and subjective well-being. *American Economic Review, 106*(12), 3869–3897.

BLANCHFLOWER, David G. & OSWALD, Andrew J. (2004). Well-being over time in Britain and the USA. *Journal of Public Economics, 88*(7–8), 1359–1386.

BLANCHFLOWER, D. G., OSWALD, A. J., & STEWART-BROWN, S. (2013). Is psychological well-being linked to the consumption of fruit and vegetables? *Social Indicators Research, 114*(3), 785–801.

BENJAMIN, Daniel J., HEFFETZ, Ori, KIMBALL, Miles S. & REES-JONES, Alex (2012). What do you think would make you happier? What do you think you would choose? *American Economic Review, 102*(5): 2083–2110.

BENJAMIN, Daniel J., HEFFETZ, Ori, KIMBALL, Miles S. & REES-JONES, Alex. (2014). Can Marginal Rates of Substitution Be Inferred from Happiness Data? Evidence from Residency Choices. *American Economic Review, 104*(11), 3498–3528.

BROWN, N. J. L. & ROHRER, J. M. (2020). Easy as (Happiness) Pie? A critical evaluation of a popular model of the determinants of well-being. *Journal of Happiness Studies 21*(4): 1285–1301. Available at: https://doi.org/10.1007/s10902-019-00128-4.

CARRILLO, A., ETCHEMENDY, E. & BAÑOS, R.M. (2020). My Best Self in the Past, Present or Future: Results of Two Randomized Controlled Trials. *Journal of Happiness Studies.* https://doi.org/10.1007/s10902-020-00259-z.

CHENG, Terence C., POWDTHAVEEE, Nattavudh, & OSWALD, Andrew J. (2017). Longitudinal evidence for a midlife nadir in human well-being: Results from four data sets.*Economic Journal, 127*(599), 126–142.

CLARK, Andrew E. (2010). Work, jobs, and well-being across the millennium. In E. Diener, J. F. Helliwell, & D. Kahneman (Eds.), *International Differences in Well-being* (pp. 436–468). Oxford University Press.

CLARK, Andrew E., SENIK, Claudia, eds. (2014). *Happiness and Economic Growth: Lessons from Developing Countries.* Oxford University Press.

CLARK, A. E., FLÈCHE, S., LAYARD, R., POWDTHAVEE, N.,& WARD, G. (2018). *The Origins of Happiness: The Science of Well-Being over the Life Course.* Princeton University Press.

DIENER, E., LUCAS, R. E., & OISHI, S. (2018). Advances and open questions in the science of subjective well-being. *Collabra: Psychology, 4*(1), 15. DOI: https://doi.org/10.1525/collab ra.115.

DIENEER, Ed., KAHNEMAN, Daniel., & HELLIWELL, John, F. (2010). *International Differences in Well-Being.* Oxford: Oxford University Press.

DIENER, Ed & TAY, Louis (2017). A scientific review of the remarkable benefits of happiness for successful and healthy living. In *Happiness Transforming the Development Landscape* (pp. 90–117). The Centre for Bhutan Studies and GNH.

DIMARIA, C. H., PERONI, C., & SARRACINO, F. (2020). Happiness Matters: Productivity Gains from Subjective Well-Being. *Journal of Happiness Studies, 21*, 139–160. https://doi.org/10.1007/s10902-019-00074-1.

DOMINKO, M., & VERBIČ, M. (2019). The Economics of Subjective Well-Being: A Bibliometric Analysis. *Journal of Happiness Studies, 20*(6), 1973–1994. https://doi.org/10.1007/s10902-018-0022-z.

FREY, Bruno S. & STUTZER, Alois. (2002). *Happiness and Economics: How the Economy and Institutions Affect Well-Being.* Princeton University Press.

FREY, Bruno S. (2018). Psychological influences on happiness. In FREY, Bruno S., and Alois STUTZER. *Economics of Happiness.* Springer, Cham., pp. 25–27.

GRAHAM, Carol (2012). *The Pursuit of Happiness: An Economy of Well-Being.* Brookings Institution Press.

GRAHAM, Carol. (2017). Happiness and economics: Insights for policy from the new "science" of well-being. *Journal of Behavioral Economics for Policy, 1*(1), 69–72.

HELLIWELL, John F. (2018). What's special about happiness as a social indicator? *Social Indicators Research, 135.3* (2018): 965–968.

KAHNEMAN, Daniel, DIENER, Ed & SCHWARZ, Norbert (Eds.) (1999).*Well-Being: The Foundations of Hedonic Psychology.* New York, NY, US: Russell Sage Foundation.

LIU, Y., LIU, J. C., LIN, M., et al. (2020). Participation of senior citizens in somatosensory games: A correlation between the willingness to exercise and happiness. *J Ambient Intell Human Comput.* https://doi.org/10.1007/s12652-020-01918-y.

LOVEDAY, P.M., LOVELL, G. P., & JONES, C.M. (2018). The best possible selves intervention: A review of the literature to evaluate efficacy and guide future research. *Journal of Happiness Studies, 19*, 607–628. https://doi.org/10.1007/s10902-016-9824-z.

LUNA-AROCAS, R., & DANVILA-DEL-VALLE, I. (2020). Does positive wellbeing predict job performance three months later? *Applied Research Quality Life.* https://doi.org/10.1007/s11482-020-09835-0.

LYKKEN, David & TELLEGEN, Auke. (1996). Happiness is a stochastic phenomenon. *Psychological Science, 7*(3), 186–189.

LYUBOMIRSKY, S., KING, L., & DIENER, E. (2005). The benefits of frequent positive affect: Does happiness lead to success? *Psychological Bulletin, 131*, 803–855.

LYUBOMIRSKY, Sonja & LAYOUS, Kristin. (2013). How do simple positive activities increase well-being? *Psychological Science, 22*, 57–62.

MINKOV, Michael & BOND, Michael (2017). A Genetic Component to National Differences in Happiness. *Journal of Happiness Studies, 18*(2): 321–340.

OSWALD, Andrew J. & WU, Stephen. (2010). Objective confirmation of subjective measures of human well-being: Evidence from the USA. *Science, 327*(5965), 576–579.

ROWLAND, Lee, CURRY, Oliver Scott (2018). A range of kindness activities boost happiness. *Journal of Social Psychology*, just-accepted (2018).

RUCH, W. F., HOFMANN, J., RUSCH, S., & STOLZ, H. (2018). Training the sense of humor with the 7 Humor Habits Program and satisfaction with life. *Humor, 31*(2), 287–309.

SCHMITT, M. T., AKNIN, L. B., AXEN, J., & SCHWOM, R. (2017). Unpacking the relationships between pro-environmental behavior, life satisfaction, and perceived ecological threat. *Ecological Economics, 143*, 130–140.

VEENHOVEN, Ruut (1984). *Conditions of Happiness*. Dordrecht: Kluwer Academic.

VEENHOVEN, Ruut. (2017). Greater happiness for a greater number: Did the promise of enlightenment come true? *Social Indicators Research, 130*(1), 9–25.

WANG, Erda and KANG, Nannan. (2018). Does life satisfaction matter for pro-environmental behavior? Empirical evidence from China General Social Survey. *Quality & Quantity*, 1–21.

Contents

1	**What is Happiness? Why is Happiness Important?**	1
	1.1 What is Happiness?	1
	1.2 Why is Happiness Important?	9
	References	11
2	**Happiness Versus Preference**	15
	References	23
3	**Some Conceptual Mistakes About Happiness**	25
	3.1 Why Do We Have Happiness?	25
	3.2 Common Mistakes About Happiness	27
	References	30
4	**Happiness or Life Satisfaction?**	33
	References	38
5	**Happiness as the Only Intrinsic Value**	41
	5.1 Happiness as the Only Intrinsic Value	41
	5.2 Answering Some Objections	47
	5.3 Rejecting Kant's Categorical Imperatives	51
	5.4 A Critique of Rawls	54
	References	56
6	**Happiness Measurability and Interpersonal Comparability**	59
	6.1 Happiness is Cardinally Measurable and Interpersonally Comparable	59
	6.2 How Could the Measurement of Happiness be Improved?	63
	References	67
7	**Does Money Buy Happiness?**	71
	References	75

8	**Environmentally Responsible Happy Nation Index: A Proposed National Success Indicator**		79
	8.1 Introduction		79
	8.2 Revising the Measurement of Happy Life Years		81
	8.3 Towards an International Acceptable National Success Indicator		82
	8.4 Estimating the Environmentally Responsible Happy Nation Index		84
	8.5 Concluding Remarks		85
	References		87
9	**Age and Happiness**		91
	9.1 The U-shape Relation of Age and Happiness		91
	9.2 The Delay in Sleep/wake Cycles of Teenagers: Ultimate Reason and Implications		93
	9.3 Chapter Appendix. Methodology		95
	References		96
10	**Factors Affecting Happiness**		99
	10.1 Maslow's Hierarchy of Needs		99
	10.2 The Four F's of Happiness		100
	10.3 Important Factors at the Social Level		105
	References		109
11	**How Do You Increase Your Happiness?**		115
	References		121
12	**Stimulating Our Brains and Transforming Our Selves**		125
	12.1 Stimulating the Pleasure Centers in Our Brains		125
	12.2 Genetic Engineering and Our Own Transformation		129
	References		130
13	**The East-Asian Happiness Gap: Causes and Implications**		133
	13.1 The East-Asian Happiness Gap		133
	13.2 Some Reflections		135
		13.2.1 Why Still the Rat-Race for Money?	136
		13.2.2 The East Asian Happiness Gap: Its Causes	136
	13.3 Some Implications		140
	References		141
14	**Implications for Public Policy**		145
	References		150
15	**A Case for Higher Public Spending**		153
	15.1 Economists Overestimate the Costs of Public Spending		154
	15.2 Specific Areas of Deficient Public Spending		157
	15.3 Concluding Remarks		158
	References		159

16 Animal Welfare: Beyond Human Happiness 161
   References 166

Appendix A: Resolving Some Moral Philosophical Controversies 167

Appendix B: Happiness as the Only Intrinsic Value: Further Opposing Arguments Considered 169

Appendix C: The Necessity of Cardinal Welfare for Rational Agents/Organisms 173

Appendix D: A Problem in Happiness Measurement 175

Appendix E: A Solution of the Moral Philosophical Problem of Optimal Population Size 177

References 179

About the Author

Yew-Kwang Ng is an emeritus professor with Monash University after serving there for nearly four decades. He has also been a Special Chair Professor at the School of Economics, Fudan University, Shanghai. He is in the Advisory Board of the Global Priorities Institute at Oxford University [https://globalprioritiesinstitute.org/about-us/.] and was invited to deliver the inaugural Atkinson Memorial Lecture in 2018, at Oxford University [published as a keynote paper in *Global Policy* 2019]. He has published more than two dozen books and three hundred refereed papers in scholarly journals, including seven single-authored papers in the top *American Economic Review*, and a single-authored paper in *Journal of Political Economy* (also one of the top 5 in economics) while an undergraduate student without supervision. His academic papers include more than two dozen on happiness and many more on the related environmental and welfare economics. He has also published many refereed papers in leading journals in philosophy and psychology. Prof. Ng has received many awards including the top award (Distinguished Fellow) of the Economic Society of Australia in 2007. e-mail: ykng@fudan.edu.cn

Chapter 1
What is Happiness? Why is Happiness Important?

Abstract The (net) happiness (or welfare) of an individual is the excess of her positive affective feelings over negative ones. This subjective definition of happiness is more consistent with common usage and analytically more useful. Over the past century or so, both psychology and economics has gone through the anti-subjectivism revolution (behaviorism in psychology and ordinalism in economics) but has come back to largely accept subjectivism (cognitive psychology and recent interest of economists on happiness issues).

1.1 What is Happiness?

Different people attain happiness in different ways. Some enjoy reading; some seldom open a book. Some enjoy spending money; some enjoy owning wealth; others enjoy non-material pursuits. Everyone wants to be happy. However, what is happiness?

A person is seldom very happy or very unhappy. Kwang may be enjoying the music that he has been listening to all-day while working and also enjoying most of the work he is doing. However, he also feels a little tired late in the afternoon after working for seven hours. (So he almost never works at night as it decreases his happiness.) As a biological organism, we feel good eating fresh and nutritious food when hungry. This clearly has survival value. Thus, contrary to the pure subjectivist, happiness is not completely subjective. The nice or bad feelings are subjective in the sense that it is felt by a person subjectively. However, they do have a substantial objective basis, although this might be shaped by the different experiences of different persons.

We feel bad when we are sick; virtually all others are like this, given the biological need for survival. If someone enjoyed being sick, he would get ill more often and have a lower chance of survival. His genes would not be passed on as successfully. In time, such genes would cease to exist. Hence, no one derives positive feelings from sickness. Thus, we can be quite confident that sickness makes the individual feel bad. This is so despite the belief by Lu Xun (鲁迅 1881–1936), a very famous Chinese writer in the first half of the twentieth century, who claimed that a small

© The Author(s) 2022
Y.-K. Ng, *Happiness—Concept, Measurement and Promotion*,
https://doi.org/10.1007/978-981-33-4972-8_1

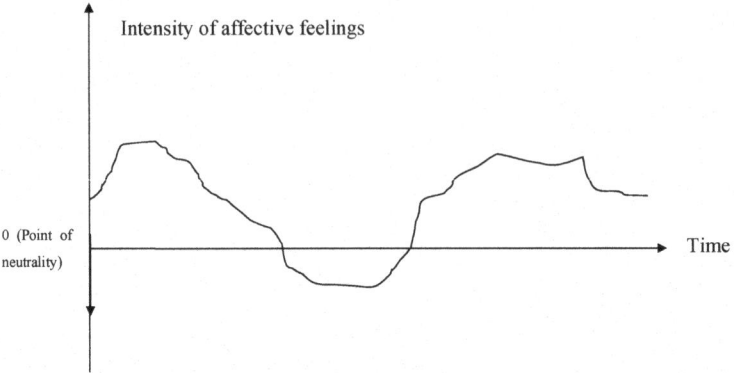

Fig. 1.1 Amount of happiness illustrated

sickness is a blessing as it allows the person enjoyment from a few days off work. The poor old Lu Xun must be very overworked!

The (net) happiness of an individual over any period of time is their nice feelings (positive affective feelings, as the psychologist calls it) less their bad (negative) feelings over that period, with both types of feelings weighted by their intensities and duration. This is a subjective conception of happiness and needs some explanation. Anyone must be capable of feeling to have happiness. Stone, water, and almost certainly, all plants, do not have happiness. Only affective feelings are included, and these are the feelings that the individual cares for positively or negatively, or that make them feel good or bad. One may visually feel the difference in the color of a book. However, if they do not care which color it is, their feeling of color here is not affective. All affective feelings are included, including the more basic good and bad feelings of smell, taste, sight, etc. and the more spiritual or sophisticated feelings of proudness, delight, shame, worry, distress, etc.

The degrees or intensities of positive or negative affective feelings of an individual over a given period of time may be represented by a curve such as the one in Fig. 1.1. Then, the amount of (net) happiness this individual enjoys over this period is given by the areas bounded by this curve above the line of neutrality minus the areas below this line. This is what I view as my happiness (over a given time interval) and I believe that I am representative of most people in this respect. This is also the concept of (objective) happiness preferred by Kahneman (1999) and sophisticatedly argued for and analysed by Kahneman et al. (1997).[1]

---

[1] For discussions of the various concepts of happiness, see, e.g. Veenhoven (1984, 2000), Kim-Prieto et al. (2005), Brülde (2007), Haybron (2007). The subjective concept I use is what philosophers called the hedonistic theory or what Haybron (2000) calls 'psychological happiness'. This is distinct from the 'prudential happiness' (or 'eudaimonic') and differs from the concept of happiness as life satisfaction itself or something similar, e.g. 'happiness as involving the realizing of global desires, a life plan, requires a level of rationality to develop' (Chekola 2007, p. 67). It is a pure affective view, a mental-state concept, and internalist (*in* your head/mind). Using 'happiness' in this sense is most consistent with the common usage of the term. For the various concepts of happiness, see Mulnix

1.1 What is Happiness?

This affective or subjective definition of happiness is called 'hedonic' in philosophy. However, for the general public, the term hedonism has a tendency to be mistakenly interpreted as being exclusively or excessively concerned with current pleasure such as to disregard the future or others. Thus, I try to avoid using 'hedonic'. If properly interpreted in its philosophical sense, there is nothing wrong with hedonism. What is wrong is harming others, not enjoying oneself.

Happiness is the most direct word and most commonly used. The meaning of 'happiness' is clear and precise and misunderstanding is minimal. 'Well-being' could be taken to be a variety of meanings, including physical well-being or economic well-being. Even if an additional adjective is added to become 'subjective well-being', it is still less precise than 'happiness'.[2] It could still mean either overall happiness or the more psychiatric sense of being free from mental illness. While 'life satisfaction' is also quite comprehensive and clear in meaning, it suffers from two fundamental problems as discussed in Chap. 4. Thus, I strongly prefer to use the terminology of 'happiness' for the concept discussed above.

Different types of feelings may be qualitatively different; beautiful sights are different from delicious tastes. However, in principle, we have no difficulty in comparing different types of feelings in terms of their quantitative significance. True, in practice, it may be difficult to compare the happiness significance of pushpins versus poetry. We may not have enough information regarding how many people really enjoy poetry and to what extent, etc. However, this is a matter of inadequate information, not incomparability in principle. As for myself, I have no difficulty in saying that I would give up pushpins rather than give up poetry (On the well-being effects of practicing poetry, see Croom 2015).

Of course, we care and/or should care about things other than our own feelings, such as the feelings of others, moral principles, etc. These relate to the happiness of others and the happiness of ourselves and others in the future. For the happiness of an individual in a given period, it consists of and only of their positive and negative feelings, as described above.

This does not mean that, for any given period, an individual only cares about or just maximizes their happiness in this period. Obviously, they take account of the effects on their future happiness. It also does not mean they maximize their own happiness only. Not only do I derive happiness by helping others to be happy (by writing this book, for example), I (and any other person) may also be prepared to sacrifice a little of our own happiness if the happiness of others may be increased substantially (more on this in Chap. 2).

---

and Mulnix (2015), Clark et al. (2018), Diener et al. (2018), Etzioni (2018), Helliwell (2018), Myers and Diener (2018) (SWB or happiness includes not just narrow sense of pleasure but all positive affective feelings like 'contentment, delight, ecstasy, elation, enjoyment, euphoria, exhilaration, exultation, gladness, gratification, gratitude, joy, liking, love, relief, satisfaction, Schadenfreude, tranquility, and so on' Moore 2013).

[2] See Diener et al. (2003) on the concept of subjective well-being.

Our definition of happiness here is purely subjective. Many scholars do not subscribe to this concept, based on a variety of grounds, which are all unacceptable in my view. Here, let us discuss just two main (somewhat interrelated) grounds for diverging from, or qualifying the purely subjective definition.

First, from Aristotle to Etzioni (2018), many knowledgeable scholars require, on top of the component of subjective affective feelings, some consistency with morality to qualify for happiness or eudaimonia. In my view, this unnecessarily confuses the two very different concepts. Being happy and being moral are two quite different concepts. One may be happy without being moral and one may be moral without being happy. Lumping the two together leads to confusion. It may be socially very desirable for us to encourage people to be moral, and/or convince them that one important way to be happy is to be moral, etc., but the two are conceptually very distinct. Essentially, to be immoral is to cause unnecessary unhappiness or reduction in happiness on others. We should use happiness to define morality, not use morality to define happiness. This latter is standing things on their head, and will likely lead to unclear thinking.[3]

Examining the *hedonic* and *eudaimonic* well-being indicators in a nationally representative longitudinal study of US adults, Pancheva et al. (2020, Abstract) show that 'the two accounts largely converged with about 70% of the sample observations registering high/low scores in both well-being dimensions'. Moreover, for the minority (30%) of divergent patterns, they 'revealed substantial changes over a 10-year period with respondents registering low *hedonic*/high *eudaimonic* well-being at time t having greater chances of upward movement toward improved well-being compared to individuals who experienced high *hedonic*/low *eudaimonic* levels in the first time period'. This supports our position that if account is taken of the effects in the future and on others, only hedonic happiness needs be taken into account.

If we view Aristotle's eudaimon as 'an ethical doctrine that would provide guidelines for how to live' (Ryff and Singer 2008, p.15), then it may be a very good guide, especially from a social viewpoint. It may also be true that 'striving to improve one's hedonic well-being fails in its aim, whereas striving to improve one's eudaimonic functioning succeeds' (Sheldon et al. 2019). Similarly, even if a firm's ultimate aim is to maximize profits, it may be counter-productive to too directly, openly, and exclusively focus on profits in all its activities; it may be more profits-efficient to emphasize much on customer relation, employee's welfare, and even market shares. However, viewed as what is ultimately of value, non-hedonic concept of happiness is debatable. Whether it is eudaimon, self-actualization, self-autonomy, etc., if the resulting outcomes involve much more misery than happiness, such that net happiness is a huge negative sum, it is not a desirable world in the ultimate or intrinsic sense.

---

[3] Thus I find the contrast between utility and morality, as discussed in the Discussion Forum on Amitai Etzioni—Twenty years of *'The Moral Dimension: Toward a New Economics'* in *Socio-Economic Review*, 2008, 6:135–173, fails to recognize points made in this chapter and in Chap. 5, and comes across as rather suspicious, if not shallow.

1.1 What is Happiness?

To avoid misunderstanding, but at the risk of repetition, let us clarify one important point. The need to take into account the effects on others and the future does not mean that the happiness of any individual for any period has to be adjusted to take into account these indirect effects. If we required such adjustment, it would become something similar to Aristotle's eudaimon. Rather, we take at face value the unadjusted happiness of any individual in any given period as of intrinsic value. Thus, if Mr. A enjoyed his binge drinking one evening, that happy feeling was then of intrinsic value. However, if his binge drinking led to his drunk driving that killed/wounded Ms. B, the great suffering imposed on Ms. B or her big loss of future happiness should be taken into account. Such accounting may thus lead us to agree that binge drinking should be discouraged or even banned. This is justified on the bad effects on others and in the future, not based on having to adjust Mr. A's happy feelings that evening. In other words, no distinction is made between personal happiness and moral happiness (or eudaimon). Happiness is happiness. But the morality of a certain act does not depend only on the effects on the happiness of the person concerned, but also on the effects on others and on the future.

Secondly, many scholars want to add some objective component to the definition of happiness. For example, as described by Adler et al. (2017a, pp. 24–5), 'The most salient objective approach among psychologists is the 'eudaimonic', or self-realization paradigm, where well-being is construed as an on-going, dynamic process of effortful living by means of engagement in *activities* perceived as meaningful (e.g., Ryan and Deci 2001). Advocates of this approach maintain that living a life of virtue, understood as developing the valuable parts of one's human nature, or actualizing one's inherent potentials in the service of something greater, constitutes the good life for an individual (Boniwell and Henry 2007; DelleFave et al. 2011). From this perspective, positive experiences are not in themselves important for a good life, and are relevant only insofar as they involving [sic] appreciating objectively worthwhile ways of being or functioning'. Similarly, Adler et al. (2017a, p. 22) defines happiness or well-being as *'everything that makes a person's life ... goes well'* (italics original).

Some happiness researchers (e.g. Kahneman 1999; Di Tella et al. 2003; Közegi and Rabin 2008; Layard and Nickell 2005; Layard 2010) are in favour of the hedonic concept while others (e.g. Ryff 1989; Waterman 1993; Etzioni 2018) are in favour of the eudaimonic concept. The majority seem to regard both as relevant. The problem with the above 'eudaimonic', 'prudential', and/or 'objective' approach to the definition of happiness is that it confuses happiness with (objective) factors that are usually conducive to happiness and elements that are usually important for the happiness in the future and of others. To minimize violations to the common meaning of the concept of happiness, and to be consistent with the universally accepted point (again from Aristotle to Etzioni 2018) that happiness is intrinsically valuable (the controversial part is that it is also the only thing that is intrinsically valuable, ultimately speaking, a point to be discussed in Chap. 5), happiness must be subjective. However, our subjective happiness is affected by a host of objective factors. The different ways or methods we lead our lives may also have very different effects on our own health, and hence our future happiness, as well as different effects on the happiness of others. For example, a person may become happy getting drunk, but may do harm to his health (hence reducing happiness in the future) or cause harm on others by drink driving, as mentioned above.

Aristotle was probably largely right that a life of contemplation and virtue, and actualizing one's inherent nature (Delle Fave et al. 2011) is the right way to wellbeing or happiness (Norton 1976), or that the usual result of eudaimonic action is hedonic happiness (Kashdan et al. 2008). 'At the opposite end, a selfish individual who has little regard for another's welfare and is primarily, or even exclusively, concerned with the pursuit of his personal interest … will usually fail to achieve both his own happiness and that of others' (Ricard 2017, pp. 160–1). Lasting happiness is associated more with selflessness rather than self-centeredness (Dambrun and Ricard 2011). Disinterested kindness to others provides profound satisfaction (Seligman 2002); kindness activities boost happiness (Dunn et al. 2008; Aknin et al. 2012, Rowland and Curry 2018). All these wise observations and research results are very important for individuals and societies in terms of promoting a good life.

However, as the basis for the definition of happiness, they only serve to confuse. For example, they lead to such misleading assertions as 'psychological wellbeing cannot exist just in your own head: it is a combination of feeling good as well as actually having meaning, engagement, good relationships, and accomplishment' (Adler et al. 2017b, p. 122). It is simpler and clearer to regard your happiness or psychological wellbeing as just existing in your own head, but your engagement, relationships, accomplishment, etc. may affect your own future happiness and that of others.

Adler et al. (2017b, p. 123) allege that the purely hedonic concept of happiness ('just in your head') 'stumbles fatally on the fact that human beings persist in having children: couples without children are likely happier, subjectively, than childless [?!] couples [with children], and so if all humans pursued … [such] subjective happiness, the species would have died out long ago'. First, this seems to be inconsistent with the finding that 'having children increases mothers' life satisfaction and happiness' (Priebe 2020, Abstract). Even ignoring this inconsistency, the argument is clearly due to the lack of consideration of the happiness of people/children in the future. A life with children may be less happy but may be a better life as it gives rise to future people with additional happiness. Thus, if happiness in the future is not ignored, the hedonic concept of happiness does not 'stumble'.[4] It is also questionable that a life with children is less happy.[5]

True, 'Objective and subjective indicators of wellbeing are both important' (Stiglitz et al. 2010, p. 15; see also Fleurbaey and Blanchet 2013; Jorgenson 2018). However, the objective indicators are important only because: 1. They are indirect

---

[4] On the relevance of future people, especially potential future people, see Ng (1989). On the other 'stumbling' allegation based on the *Brave New World*, see Chap. 2.

[5] 'For parents who have had children due to the generosity of family policies, having children increases parent's life satisfaction by 0.33–0.41 points on a 10 point scale. This effect is significantly more pronounced when parents are over the age of 50. Yet, children's effects on life satisfaction and happiness is negative for single and full-time working parents. The positive effect of having children on life satisfaction and happiness has substantially eroded over the EVS (European Values Survey) waves which explains the reductions in the fertility rate in Europe' (Ugur 2020, Abstract).

1.1 What is Happiness?

indicators of subjective wellbeing; 2. They are important for subjective wellbeing (i.e. happiness) in the future; 3. They are important for the subjective wellbeing of others. One of the reasons the second factor may be important maybe because they contribute to the prevention of government's manipulation of 'people's preferences and/or knowledge' (Unanue 2017, p. 75). Similar to this possible usefulness of objective indicators of happiness, the 'operational definition' of happiness (Thin et al. 2017, p. 40) may also be useful. However, properly understood, it should be 'operational indicators', not definitions of happiness. Also similarly, such factors as capabilities, functioning, flourishing, etc. (see, e.g. Hasan 2019) are important also, ultimately speaking, only for their contributions to welfare or happiness.

Consider: 'Sen (1999, p. 14) provides some more realistic cases that may have significant relevance to public policy. Sen thinks hedonism is problematic because '[a] person who is ill-fed, undernourished, unsheltered and ill can still be high up in the scale of happiness or desire-fulfillment if he or she has learned to have realistic desires and to take pleasure in small mercies.' If such a person can be said to be doing well, then there seems to be something problematic about hedonism. Our tendency is to say that person has adapted as best as she can to poor life circumstances, and she is making the best of a bad situation, but that does not mean she is doing well: The destitute thrown into beggary, the vulnerable landless labourer precariously surviving at the edge of subsistence, the over-worked domestic servant working around the clock, the subdued and subjugated housewife reconciled to her role and her fate, all tend to come to terms with their respective predicaments. (p. 15)' (Hersch 2018, p. 2234). In my view, such cases may well be very undesirable; however, this is so because they tend to reduce happiness in the long run. Taking account of effects in the future and on others will account for them. On the other hand, if they do not [unlikely though] reduce happiness in the long run, they are not bad.

Despite the above explanations, some people may still prefer to have a different conception of happiness. For example, consider two hypothetical scholars who both died in an air crash at the same age. Madam A suffered from debilitating illness and a broken family throughout much of her life, leading to her undergoing enormous pain and distress. However, working long and exhausting hours, she made important breakthroughs in knowledge and was awarded a Nobel prize just before her death. Though she died happy, her unhappiness throughout her whole life clearly outweighs her final happiness for a few days. Mr. B was a healthy and happily married man who enjoyed life a lot. He also enjoyed his work and performed satisfactorily. Just before his death, he learned that his expected promotion did not go through as it was found that his only major contribution was contained in another publication years before his. He died unhappy and his career was not a very successful one. However, his final unhappiness for a few days is far exceeded by his high level of happiness for a long time.

According to our conception of happiness, Madam A had an unhappy life while Mr. B had a happy one. However, according to some other conception of happiness (which emphasizes final satisfaction with one's life), A had a happy life and B had an unhappy one. Moreover, some, if not many, people may prefer to have a life like A's to one like B's. Several issues are involved here.

To simplify from the complication of interest earnings from savings, assume a society with zero interest rate and zero inflation rate. Consider two persons similar in all aspects except that X had a high annual income and consumption level ($80,000) during the first half of his life which was unexpectedly halved in the second half of life. In contrast, Y started with half the initial level of X's (i.e. $40,000) for the first half of his life but the level was unexpectedly doubled for the second half. Though their income and consumption over the whole life are the same, Y probably had a happier life, provided that the level of $40,000 per annum was not so low as to make him malnourished. (Malnourishment in the first half may be worse than that in the second half as it could affect one's health for both halves.) Subject to this proviso, most people also prefer to be in the situation of Y than X. When one has been accustomed to a high level of consumption, one needs a high level to be happy. Thus, subject to the absence of health-damaging under-consumption, it is better to have a profile of increasing consumption level than one that is decreasing. However, this consideration does not apply to the case of Madam A versus Mr. B where the profiles are already stated in terms of happiness, not in terms of consumption.

Many people may have faulty telescopic faculty so as not to make full allowance for the future, as believed by Pigou (1912, 1929, 1932, p. 25), a well-known economist early in the twentieth century. When one looks backward in time, events far back may also appear less important. But this is a similar mistake as having a faulty telescopic faculty.

Madam A had a more successful life than Mr. B who had a happier life. The difference is due to A's much higher contribution to knowledge which, presumably, would make others happier. Madam A may also have a higher life satisfaction than B, at least at the end, but this is still not a happier life. A may prefer to have her unhappy life over B's happy life. She may rationally have this preference if she believed that her contribution to knowledge would make others happier and if she cared for the happiness of others. This care may make life satisfaction (which is more likely affected by one's contribution to others) differ from the happiness of the same person, as will be discussed further in Chap. 4.

True, despite the above explanations, some people may still opt to use a somewhat different conception of happiness than the one we define above. However, the fact that momentary experience sampling (Csikszentmihalyi and Hunter 2003) of happiness and fatigue is predictive of cardiovascular disease progression, while overall evaluation of life is not so predictive (Karmarck et al. 2007), support both the use of momentary experience sampling as a method of measuring happiness and our definition of happiness above. Moreover, most people will agree that the good and bad feelings one has are important in affecting whether one is happy or not, even if not exclusively. Thus, one does not have to agree with our conception of happiness completely to find the rest of this book interesting and important.

In addition to the above two points, many scholars (including Sumner 1996; Chekola 2007; Adler 2017b) want to include some cognitive element into happiness or subjective well-being (SWB). Some define SWB as being inclusive of both affective happiness and cognitive life satisfaction. I find this confusing, if not also misleading. Using happiness, welfare and SWB as synonymous and defined in the affective sense as discussed above, is most consistent with the common usage and most useful analytically. Then, usually one's life satisfaction (defined cognitively) may largely be affected by one's own happiness, but also by one's belief in contribution to society (ultimately and rationally, should be to happiness). Then, it is at least conceptually possible for most or even all individuals in a society to be unhappy (net happiness being negative) and yet still have high life satisfaction, as discussed in more detail in Chap. 4. This may be due to each believing that she has made huge contributions to the happiness of others. Yet, due to imperfect knowledge or misfortunes, the believed (perhaps mistakenly) contributions did not really materialize into happiness for most individuals. At least in outcome, such a society of unhappy individuals is miserable, despite high life satisfaction. Life satisfaction is not meaningless and may be useful for certain purposes, including the potential to affect happiness in the future. Happiness and life satisfaction also tend to be mutually reinforcing. However, ultimately, it is happiness that is of intrinsic value. Thus, I prefer to focus mainly on happiness, especially when the two differ, as discussed further in the next section and Chap. 4.

1.2 Why is Happiness Important?

Over the past century or more, psychology has gone through at least three important phases of subjectivism, behaviorism, and cognitivism. Classical psychologists spoke of mind, consciousness, and used introspection in their analysis. Then came the Watson-Skinner behaviorist revolution which prohibited the analysis of anything subjective: only actual behaviors were the proper subject matter of psychology. This allowed psychology to make huge advances in becoming more scientific, but concomitantly caused some to feel that it had 'gone out of its mind…and lost all consciousness' (Chomsky 1959, p. 29). The reaction against the excesses of behaviorism resulted in the cognitive revolution which has been prevalent for the past few decades, and which has made much headway.

Economics has gone through similar phases. Older economists (since the Neoclassical revolution in the nineteen century) used more subjective terms like satisfaction, marginal utility, and even happiness, pleasure, and pain. After the indifference-curve or ordinalism revolution in the 1930s, modern economists are very adverse to the more subjective concepts and very hostile to cardinal utility and interpersonal comparisons of utility. (See Kaminitz 2018 on the histories and approaches on this by economists and psychologists.) They prefer to use the more objective concepts like preference and choice. In a very important sense, these changes represent an important methodological advance, making economic analysis to be based on more objective grounds. However, the change or correction has been carried into excess, making economics unable to tackle many important problems, divorced from fundamental concepts, and even misleading. In my view, while we should prefer to use more objective concepts when they are sufficient, we should not shy away from the more subjective concepts and even their interpersonal comparison when they are needed.

Perhaps we may date the commencement of the subjectivist counter-revolution to the dominance of objectivism/ordinalism in economics at 1997, with the appearance of three papers (Oswald 1997; Frank 1997; Ng 1997) on happiness in *Economic Journal*, with Easterlin (1974) as the earliest forerunner. In the last 2–3 decades, many top journals in economics have published papers on happiness studies and economists are less reluctant to speak in terms of subjective concepts including happiness, including its cardinal measurability and interpersonal comparability.

Happiness is more important than the objective concepts of choice, preference and income (especially if narrowly interpreted and eschewing cardinal utility and interpersonal comparison, as is the usual practice in modern economics) for at least two reasons. First, happiness is the ultimate objective of most, if not all people (more on this in Chap. 5). We want money (or anything else) only as a means to increase our happiness. If having more money does not substantially increase our happiness (Chap. 7), then money is not very important, but happiness is.

Secondly, for economically advanced countries (the number of which is increasing) there is evidence suggesting that, for the whole of society, and in the long run (in real purchasing power terms), money does not buy happiness, or at least not much (Easterlin 1974; Veenhoven 1984; Argyle and Martin 1991, p. 80; Oswald 1997; Asadullah et al. 2018; Cheng et al. 2018; Luo et al. 2018). This is known as the Easterlin paradox of unhappy growth, the failure of money or economic growth to increase happiness (For the sister paradox of happy stagnation for Japan in the last three decades, see Chap. 13). The reasons are not difficult to see. Once the basic necessities and comforts of life are adequate, further consumption can actually make us worse off due to problems like excessive fat and cholesterol and stress. Our ways to increase happiness further then take on the largely competitive forms like attempting to keep up with or surpassing the Joneses. From a social viewpoint, such competition is a pure waste (Frank 1997). On top of this, production and consumption to sustain the competition continue to impose substantial environmental costs, making economic growth quite possibly happiness-decreasing (Ng and Wang 1993, and Chap. 7). To avoid this sad outcome, a case can be made for *increasing* public spending (contrary to the currently popular view against public expenditures among economists) to safeguard the environment and to engage in research and development that will increase welfare (Ng 2003*)*. This is especially so since relative-income effects makes the traditional estimate of optimal public spending sub-optimal (Ng 1987a). As the schoolmates of one's child all receive expensive birthday gifts, one feels the need to give as expensive gifts. Thus, the perceived importance of private expenditures is inflated relative to that of public spending (Ng 2003 and Chaps. 14 and 15).

The return of both psychology and economics to largely accept subjectivism is unavoidable and much to be welcome. Happiness is the ultimate and only intrinsic value (Chap. 5) and it is subjective. The great British economist Arthur Pigou (1922) regarded the study of economics (and arguably other studies as well, though we should not insist on immediate effects) should be mainly for bearing fruits, not just shedding lights (though shedding lights itself is a kind of fruit). Happiness is the ultimate fruit.

References

ADLER, Alejandro, BONIWELL, Ilona, GIBSON, Evelyn, METZ, Thaddeus, SELIGMAN, Martin, UCHIDA, Yukiko & XING, Zhanjun (2017a). Definitions of terms. In *Happiness Transforming the Development Landscape*, pp. 21–38, The Centre for Bhutan Studies and GNH.

ADLER, Alejandro, UNANUE, Wenceslao, OSIN, Evgeny, RICARD, Matthieu, ALKIRE, Sabina & SELIGMAN, Martin (2017b). Psychological wellbeing. In *Happiness Transforming the Development Landscape*, pp. 118–155), The Centre for Bhutan Studies and GNH.

AEGYLE, M., & MARTIN, M. (1991). The psychological causes of happiness. In STRACK, F., ARGYLE, M., & SCHWARZ, N. (Eds.), *Subjective well-being. An interdisciplinary perspective*, pp. 77–100, Oxford: Pergamon Press.

AKNIN, L. B., HAMLIN, J. K., & DUNN, E. W. (2012). Giving leads to happiness in young children. *PLoS One*, 7(6), e39211.

ASADULLAH, M. N., XIAO, S., & YEOH, E. (2018). Subjective well-being in China, 2005–2010: The role of relative income, gender, and location. *China Economic Review*, 48, 83–101.

BONIWELL, Ilona & HENRY, Jane (2007). Developing conceptions of well-being. *Social Psychology Review*, 9: 3–18.

BRÜLDE, Bengt (2007). Happiness and the good life. Introduction and conceptual framework. *Journal of Happiness Studies*, 8(1): 1–14.

CHEKOLA, Mark (2007). Happiness, rationality, autonomy and the good life. *Journal of Happiness Studies*, 8(1): 51–78.

CHENG, H., CHEN, C., LI, D., & YU, H. (2018). The mystery of Chinese people's happiness. *Journal of Happiness Studies*, 19(7), 2095–2114.

CHOMSKY, N. (1959). A review of BF Skinner's Verbal Behavior. *Language*, 35(1), 26–58.

CLARK, A. E., FLÈCHE, S., LAYARD, R., POWDTHAVEE, N., & WARD, G. (2018). *The Origins of Happiness: The Science of Well-Being over the Life Course*, Princeton University Press.

CROOM, A. M. (2015). The practice of poetry and the psychology of well-being. *Journal of Poetry Therapy*, 28, 21–41.

CSIKSZENTMIHALYI, Mihaly & HUNTER, Jeremy (2003). Happiness in everyday life: The uses of experience sampling. *Journal of Happiness Studies*, 4: 185–199.

DAMBRUN, Michaël & RICARD, Matthieu (2011). Self-centeredness and selflessness: A theory of self-based psychological functioning and its consequences for happiness. *Review of General Psychology*, 15(2): 138–157.

DELLE FAVE, Antonella, MASSIMINI, Fausto & BASSI, Marta (2011).Hedonism and eudaimonism in positive psychology. In A. DelleFave (Eds.) *Psychological Selection and Optimal Experience across Cultures. Cross-Cultural Advancements in Positive Psychology*, 2: 3–18.New York: Springer.

DI TELLA, R., MACCULLOCH, R., OSWALD, A. (2003). "The Macroeconomics of Happiness", *Review of Economics and Statistics*, 85(4): 809–827.

DIENER, E., LUCAS, R. E., & OISHI, S. (2018). Advances and open questions in the science of subjective well-being. *Collabra: Psychology*, 4(1), 15. DOI: https://doi.org/10.1525/collab ra.115.

DIENER, Ed, SCOLLON, Christie, N. & LUCAS, Richard, E. (2003). The evolving concept of subjective wellbeing: the multifaceted nature of happiness. *Advances in Cell Aging and Gerontology*, 15: 187–219.

DUNN, E. W., AKNIN, L. B., & NORTON, M. I. (2008). Spending money on others promotes happiness. *Science*, 319(5870), 1687–1688.

EASTERLIN, Richard A. (1974). Does economic growth improve the human lot? Some empirical evidence. In DAVID, Paul, & REDER, Melvin W. (eds.) *Nations and Households in Economic Growth, Essays in Honor of Moses Abramovitz*. New York: Academic Press.

ETZIONI, Amitai (2018). Happiness is the wrong metric. In *Happiness is the Wrong Metric*, pp. 3–40. Springer, Cham.

FLEURBAEY, Marc and DIDIER, BLANCHET (2013). *Beyond GDP: Measuring Welfare and Assessing Sustainability,* Oxford University Press.

FRANK, R. H. (1997). Conspicuous consumption: Money well spent? *Journal of Economic,* 107: 1832–1847.

HASAN, Hamid (2019). Confidence in subjective evaluation of human well-being in Sen's capabilities perspective, Journal of Happiness Studies, 20(1): 1–17.

HAYBRON, D. M. (2000). Two philosophical problems in the study of happiness, *Journal of Happiness Studies,* 1(2): 207–225.

HAYBRON, Daniel M. (2007). Life satisfaction, ethical reflection, and the science of happiness. *Journal of Happiness Studies,* 8: 99–138.

HELLIWELL, John F. (2018). What's special about happiness as a social indicator? *Social Indicators Research* 135.3 (2018): 965–968.

HERSCH, Gil (2018). Ignoring Easterlin: Why Easterlin's correlation findings need not matter to public policy. *Journal of Happiness Studies, 19*(8), 2225–2241.

JORGENSON, Dale W. (2018). Production and welfare: progress in economic measurement. *Journal of Economic Literature,* 61(3): 867–919.

KAHNEMAN, Daniel. (1999). Objective happiness. In D. Kahneman, E. Diener & N. Schwarz (eds.). *Well-being: The foundations of hedonic psychology* (pp. 3–25). Russell Sage Foundation.

KAHNEMAN, Daniel, WAKKER, Peter P. & SARIN, Rakesh (1997).Back to bentham? Explorations of experienced utility. *Quarterly Journal of Economics,* 112(2): 375–405.

KAMINITZ, S. C. (2018). Happiness studies and the problem of interpersonal comparisons of satisfaction: Two histories, three approaches. Journal of Happiness Studies 19(2), 423–442. https://doi.org/10.1007/s10902-016-9829-7

KARMARCK, Thomas W., MULDOON, Matthew F., SHIFFMAN, Saul S., & SUTTON-TYRRELL, Kim (2007). Experiences of demand and control during daily life are predictors of carotid atherosclerotic progression among health men. *Health Psychology,* 26: 324–332.

KASHDAN, Todd. B., BISWAS-DIENER, Robert & KING, Laura A. King, (2008). Reconsidering happiness: The costs of distinguishing between hedonics and eudaimonia. *Journal of Positive Psychology,* 3(4): 219–233.

KIM-PRIETO, Chu, DIENER, Ed, TAMIR, Maya, SCOLLON, Christie & DIENER, Marissa (2005). Integrating the diverse definitions of happiness: A time-sequential framework of subjective well-being. *Journal of Happiness Studies,* 6(3): 261–300.

KŐSZEGI, Botond & RABIN, Matthew (2008). Choices, situations, and happiness. *Journal of Public Economics,* 92(8), 1821–1832.

LAYARD, R., MAYRAZ, G. & NICKELL, S. (2010). Does relative income matter? Are the critics right? In Diener, et al. pp. 139–165.

LAYARD, Richard (2005). *Happiness: Lessons from a New Science.* New York and London: Penguin.

LUO, Yangmei, WANG, Tong, and HUANG, Xiting (2018) . Which types of income matter most for well-being in China: Absolute, relative or income aspirations? *International Journal of Psychology,* 53(3): 218–222.

MOORE, A. (2013). Hedonism. In Zalta, E. N. (Ed.), *The Stanford Encyclopedia of Philosophy.* https://www.plato.stanford.edu/archives/win2013/entries/hedonism/.

MULNIX, Jennifer W. & MULNIX, M. J. (Eds.) (2015).*Theories of Happiness: An Anthology.* Broadview Press.

MYERS, David G. and DIENER, Ed (2018). The scientific pursuit of happiness. *Perspectives on Psychological Science* 13(2): 218–225.

NG, Yew-Kwang (1987). Relative-income effects and the appropriate level of public expenditure, *Oxford Economic Papers,* 293–300.

NG, Yew-Kwang (1989). What should we do about future generations? The impossibility of Parfit's theory X. *Economics and Philosophy,* 5(2): 235–253.

NG, Yew-Kwang (1997). A case for happiness, cardinal utility, and interpersonal comparability. *Economic Journal,* 107 (445): 1848–1858.

References

NG, Yew-Kwang & LIU, Po-Ting (2003). Global environmental protection – solving the international public-good problem by empowering the United Nations through cooperation with WTO. *International Journal of Global Environmental Issues*, 3(4): 409–417.

NG, Yew-Kwang & WANG, Jianguo (1993). Relative income, aspiration, environmental quality, individual and political myopia: Why may the rat-race for material growth be welfare reducing? *Mathematical Social Sciences*, 26: 3–23.

NORTON, David L. (1976). *Personal Destinies: A Philosophy of Ethical Individualism*. Princeton University Press.

OSWALD, Andrew J. (1997).Happiness and economic performance. *The Economic Journal*, 107: 1815–1831.

PANCHEVA, M.G., RYFF, C.D. & LUCCHINI, M. (2020). An integrated look at well-being: Topological clustering of combinations and correlates of *hedonia* and *eudaimonia*. *Journal of Happiness Studies*. https://doi.org/10.1007/s10902-020-00325-6

PIGOU, Arthur C. (1912/1929/1932), *Wealth and Welfare*. Later editions (1920, 1924, 1929, 1932) assume the title *The Economics of Welfare*. London: Macmillan.

PIGOU, Arthur C. (1922), Empty economic boxes: A reply. *Economic Journal*, 32: 458–465.

PRIEBE, J. (2020). Quasi-experimental evidence for the causal link between fertility and subjective well-being. *J Popul Econ* 33, 839–882. https://doi.org/10.1007/s00148-020-00769-3

RICARD, Matthieu (2017). Altruism and happiness. In *Happiness Transforming the Development Landscape* (pp. 156–68). The Centre for Bhutan Studies and GNH.

ROWLAND, Lee, and CURRY, Oliver Scott (2018). A range of kindness activities boost happiness. *Journal of Social Psychology,* just-accepted (2018).

RYAN, Richard M. & DECI, Edward L. (2001). On happiness and human potentials: a review of research on hedonic and eudaimonic well-being. *Annual Review of Psychology, 52*, 141–166.

RYFF, Carol D. & SINGER, Burton H. (2008). Know thyself and become what you are: A eudaimonic approach to psychological well-being. *Journal of Happiness Studies*, 9:13–39.

RYFF, Carol D. (1989). Happiness is everything, or is it? Explorations on the meaning of psychological wellbeing. *Journal of Personality and Social Psychology*, 57: 1069–1081.

SELIGMAN, M. E. P. (2002) . *Authentic Happiness: Using the New Positive Psychology To realize Your Potential for Lasting Fulfillment*. New York: Free Press.

SEN, A. (1999). *Development as freedom*. New York: Borzoi.

SHELDON, K.M., CORCORAN, M. & PRENTICE, M. (2019). Pursuing eudaimonic functioning versus pursuing hedonic well-being: The first goal succeeds in its aim, Whereas the second does not. *Journal of Happiness Studies* 20(3), 919–933. https://doi.org/10.1007/s10902-018-9980-4

STIGLITZ, Joseph E., SEN, Amartya. & FITOUSI, Jean-Paul (2010). *Mismeasuring Our Lives: Why GDP Doesn't Add Up*. New York, N.Y.: New Press.

SUMNER, Leonard W. (1996). *Welfare, Happiness and Ethics*. New York: Clarendon Press.

THIN, Neil, HAYBRON, Daniel, BISWAS-DIENER, Robert, AHUVIA, Aaron & TIMSIT, Jean (2017). Desirability of sustainable happiness as a guide for public policy.In *Happiness Transforming the Development Landscape* (pp. 39–59).The Centre for Bhutan Studies and GNH.

UGUR, Z.B. (2020). Does having children bring life satisfaction in Europe?. *Journal of Happiness Studies* 21(4), 1385–1406. https://doi.org/10.1007/s10902-019-00135-5

UNANUE, Wenceslao (2017). Subjective wellbeing measures to inform public policies. *Happiness*, The Centre for Bhutan Studies and GNH,60.

VEENHOVEN, Ruut (1984). *Conditions of Happiness*. Dordrecht: Kluwer Academic.

VEENHOVEN, Ruut (2000). The four qualities of life: Ordering concepts and measures of the good life. *Journal of Happiness Studies*, 1: 1–39.

WATERMAN, Alan S. (1993). Two conceptions of happiness: Contrasts of personal expressiveness (eudaimonia) and hedonic enjoyment. *Journal of Personality and Social Psychology*, 64: 678–691.

Open Access This chapter is licensed under the terms of the Creative Commons Attribution 4.0 International License (http://creativecommons.org/licensediverse definition/by/4.0/), which permits use, sharing, adaptation, distribution and reproduction in any medium or format, as long as you give appropriate credit to the original author(s) and the source, provide a link to the Creative Commons license and indicate if changes were made.

The images or other third party material in this chapter are included in the chapter's Creative Commons license, unless indicated otherwise in a credit line to the material. If material is not included in the chapter's Creative Commons license and your intended use is not permitted by statutory regulation or exceeds the permitted use, you will need to obtain permission directly from the copyright holder.

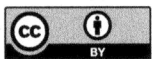

Chapter 2
Happiness Versus Preference

Abstract The preference of an individual may differ from her happiness due to imperfect information, a true concern for the welfare of others (non-affective altruism), and imperfect rationality. In some exceptional circumstances, such as the traditional Chinese custom of giving the deceased parent a decent burial and not to disturb them by re-burial, some measures (like banning slavery and using a cemetery for essential developments) may improve social welfare, even if against the preferences of most, and perhaps all, people.

I define happiness, subjective well-being, and welfare of an individual as essentially equivalent terms, with only two minor differences in usage. First, we tend to use 'happiness' to refer to the **current** feeling. If I see you singing and dancing gladly, I tend to say that you are happy now. If I know that you are healthy and have a loving spouse, nice children, good income, etc., I tend to conclude that your welfare must be high, because you will likely be happy for a **long** time. Second, we tend to use 'happy', 'happiness' in a less formal way and 'subjective well-being' and 'welfare' in a more formal way. For example, as mentioned by Diener and Tay (2017, p. 90), 'Subjective wellbeing, often called "happiness" in layperson terminology, refers to peoples' sense of wellness in their lives'. If we ignore the formality in usage and holding the time period as given, I find that my happiness, subjective well-being, and welfare must be exactly identical. If a person is unhappy through her whole life, her welfare cannot be high; her subjective well-being cannot be positive.

Since most, if not all individuals care much about their own welfare, preference and welfare normally go together (Benjamin et al. 2012). However, the preference of an individual may differ from her happiness or welfare for the following three reasons.

First, preference may differ from welfare due to ignorance and imperfect foresight. While an individual may prefer x to y, believing he will be better off in x than in y, it may turn out to be the other way around. This is the question of an *ex-ante* estimate versus *ex-post* welfare. While the *ex-ante* concept is relevant for explaining behavior, it is the *ex-post* one which is the actual welfare.

Second, the preference of an individual may not only be affected by her own welfare but may also be affected by her consideration for the welfare of other individuals. Thus, it is possible for a person to personally have a higher happiness level in y than in x, yet herself prefers and chooses x over y because she believes that other people are happier in x than in y. While it is true that the belief that other people are happy may make her happy, these positive feelings may not be strong enough to outweigh the loss that she has to suffer for changing from y to x. For example, a person may vote for party x, knowing that she herself will be better off with party y in government. The reason she votes for x is that she believes that the majority of the people will be much better off with x. This itself may make her *feel* better (affective altruism). However, this external benefit may not be important enough to overbalance, in terms of her subjective happiness, her personal loss, say in income, under x. She may yet vote for x due to her moral concern (non-affective altruism) for the majority. To give an even more dramatic example, consider an individual who expects to lead a very happy life. When her country is being invaded, she may volunteer for a mission which will bring her the certainty of death. The prospect of being a citizen of a conquered nation especially with the guilt conscience of failing to volunteer for the mission may not be too bright. But overall she may still expect to be fairly happy in leading such a life. Yet she chooses death for the sake of her fellow countrymen. In this case, she is not maximizing her own welfare.

Some economists have difficulty in seeing the above distinction between preference and welfare, saying that whenever an individual prefers x to y, she must be, or at least believe herself to be happier in x than in y. This difficulty completely baffles me. Clearly, a father (or mother) may sacrifice his (her) happiness for the welfare of his (her) children. I cannot see why similar sacrifices cannot be made for a friend or a relative, and further for a countryman, any human being, and finally, any sentient creature.[1]

It may be doubted that the existence of true non-affective altruism is inconsistent with Darwinian natural selection. However, as preferences are the result of both cultural and genetic inheritance, one can demonstrate that pro-social traits could have evolved under the joint influence of cultural and genetic transmission.[2]

If some readers still doubt the existence of truly non-affective altruism, they are likely to be convinced that in fact they themselves possess some degree of non-affective altruism by considering the following hypothetical choice. Like Einstein's thought experiments, such hypothetical exercises cannot be dismissed on the ground

---

[1] For some interviews with some real-life altruists, see Monroe (1996), Part I. For a survey of some evidence of true altruism, see Hoffman (1981). One type of evidence is that a person is more likely to help others when he/she is the only person around, contrary to the egoistic explanation of helping on the ground of approval gaining. Cf. Charness and Rabin (2002).

[2] As shown by Boyd and Richerson (1985), Sober and Wilson (1998), and Bowles (2000). Moreover, 'highly developed human capacities for insider-outsider distinctions and cultural uniformity within communities greatly increase the likely importance of group selection of genetically transmitted traits, and hence the evolutionary viability of group-beneficial traits' (Bowles and Gintis 2000, p. 1419). On the evolutionary basis of altruism towards one's relatives, see Hamilton (1964) and Bergstrom (1996).

of being unrealistic. Suppose that you are asked by the Devil to press either button A or B within 2 s. You know with certainty (for simplicity of comparison) that one of the following will happen depending on which button you press. Within these two seconds, you will be so preoccupied with pressing the right button such that your welfare will be zero whichever button you press. After pressing, you will lose memory of the present world and hence will not have feelings of guilt, warm-glow, or the like, related to which button you press.

- A: You will go to Bliss with a welfare level of 1,000,000 trillion units. Everyone else will go to Hell with a welfare level of minus 1,000,000 trillion units each.
- B: You will go to Bliss Minus with a welfare level of 999,999 trillion units. Everyone else will go to Niceland with a welfare level of 999 trillion units each.
- C: If you do not press either button within the 2 s, you and everyone else will go to Hell.

By construction, choosing A will maximize your welfare but most people will choose B out of non-affective altruism. If you still think that you will choose A, change Bliss Minus into a welfare level of 999,999.999 trillion units. If you still opt for A, I have to concede that you are not altruistic non-affectively. But how could you have the heart to condemn all others to Hell for a fractional increase in your own welfare? (In my view, the existence and degree of non-affective altruism marks true morality.)

Third, an individual may have irrational (or imperfectly rational) preferences. The preference of an individual is here defined as irrational if he prefers x over y despite the fact that his welfare is higher in y than in x, and his preference is unaffected by considerations of the welfare of other individuals (any sentient creature can be an individual here), or by ignorance or imperfect foresight. The definition of irrationality here is so as to make the three factors discussed here exhaustive causes of divergence between preference and welfare.

While few, if any individuals are perfectly ignorant and irrational, some degrees of ignorance (or imperfect information) and imperfect rationality clearly apply to most individuals.[3] However, some alleged irrationalities could be simply due to errors, computational limitations, and incorrect norm by the experimenters (Stanovich and West 2000). There are a number of causes that may make preferences differ from happiness other than ignorance and a concern for the welfare of others, and hence they are irrational according to our definition here. The following two (may not be completely independent) causes may both be explained, at least partly, by some biological factors (On the biological basis of social behaviour, see, e.g. Wilson 1975; Crawford & Kreps, 1998; Nicolosi and Maestrutti 2016).

First, there is a tendency for many people to discount the future too much or even to ignore it completely. This is widely noted, including by economists. For example, Pigou (1912, 1929, 1932, p. 25) called it the "*faulty telescopic faculty*", Ramsey (1928, p. 543) called it "*weakness of imagination*" about the future, and Harrod

---

[3] See Cohen (1983), Evans and Over (1996), Kahneman and Tversky (2013), Stein (1996), Igaki et al. (2019) for reviews of the relevant literature in philosophy and psychology.

(1948, p. 40) regarded it as the *"conquest of reason by passion"*. A discount on future consumption, income, and any other monetary value is rational as a dollar now can be transformed into more than a dollar in the future. A discount on future utility may still be rational if the realization of future utility is uncertain. (For healthy people, this uncertainty is usually very small per annum.) Discounting the future for more than these acceptable reasons is probably irrational. A manifestation of this irrationality is the insufficient amount of savings for old age, necessitating compulsory and heavily subsidized superannuation schemes. I came across an extreme example of such under-saving during a survey regarding how much people would be willing to save more if the rate of interest were higher (Ng 1992). The question implicitly assumed that everyone did some saving, as the answers were in terms of how many percentages more one would save. One subject declared that he did not save anything. I then asked him to change the answers to be chosen from "saving 20% more" into "saving $20 more per month". He said he could not be persuaded to save anything at whatever interest rates (500% was mentioned). He only conceded willingness to save when I said, "What if a dollar saved now will become a million dollars next year?" I was careful enough to find out that this healthy-looking young man was not expecting early death from a terminal disease or the like.

The behaviour of most other animals is largely determined by pre-programmed instincts rather than the careful calculation of the present costs versus future benefits. The storing of food by ants, the burial of nuts by squirrels, etc. are largely, if not completely, instinctive. If calculated choices are made by animals, they are largely confined to sizing up the current situation to decide the best move at the moment, like fight or flight. The ability to anticipate the rewards in the fairly distant future requires much more 'reason', 'imagination', and 'telescopic faculty' than normally cost-effective to program in most other species. However, we know that we are endowed with some such faculty. Nevertheless, since this advanced faculty is almost completely absent in most other species, it is natural to expect that it is not fully developed even in our own species. Moreover, different members of our species may be endowed with different degrees of such faculty. The existence of a significant proportion of members of our species which do not possess a full telescopic faculty is thus not surprising.

Secondly, there are the excessive temptation of pleasure (especially present pleasure vs. future costs, hence related to the preceding cause) and the powerful biological drives. After the evolution of flexible species (defined as one where the behavior of its members is not completely determined by the automatic programmed responses but also by choice), natural selection ensured that the flexible choices made were largely consistent with fitness by endowing the flexible species with the reward-penalty system. Thus, eating when hungry and mating with fertile members of the opposite sex are rewarded with pleasure, and damages to the body are penalized with pain. (This makes the flexible species also "rational" as defined in Ng 1996 which shows that complex niches favor rational species which in turn make the environment more complex, leading to a virtuous cycle that accelerates the rate of evolution. This partly explains the dramatic speed of evolution based mainly on random mutation and natural selection, a speed doubted by creationists.) On top of the *ex-post* rewards and penalties, we are also endowed with inner drives to satisfy the fitness-enhancing functions like mating. On the whole, these powerful temptations and drives work in the right direction, making us do things that both enhance our biological fitness and psychological welfare. However, since evolution is largely fitness-maximization and the welfare-enhancing aspect is only indirectly to enhance fitness, some divergence between our behavior and our welfare is unavoidable, as our behavior is not completely determined by rational calculation, but also partly by programmed inclination, including the drives. (See Ng 1995 on the divergence between fitness and welfare maximization especially with respect to the number of offspring.)

It has also been shown that, 'wanting' or preference and 'liking' or welfare are mediated by different neural systems in the brain and are psychologically dissociable from each other. In other words, an individual may prefer something without liking it or prefer something more strongly than could be justified by his liking for it, and vice versa. In particular, neural sensitization of brain dopamine systems by addictive drugs may create intense 'wanting' way beyond that which could be explained by 'liking' and the relieving of withdrawal symptoms. (See Berridge 1999 for a review.) As an example of these powerful drives, adolescent girls and boys often engage in careless sexual acts propelled by their sexual drive and the temptation of sexual pleasure, even if there is a high risk to their long-term welfare, such as in the case of unwanted pregnancies or the contraction of AIDS. While this is partly due to ignorance, the role of biological drives cannot be denied.

Consider a specific example. Suppose that a person agrees that, for choices involving risks, the correct thing to do is to maximize expected welfare (assuming no effects on the welfare of others) and also actually do so for most choices. However, for choices concerning sexual activities, he chooses x over y, although his expected welfare is lower with x than with y and he knows this to be the case. Here, x may involve having sex with many persons without clear knowledge (this knowledge is assumed to be not feasible to obtain and hence not relevant) about whether they have AIDS. His (expected) welfare-reducing choice of x may be due to his biological inclination to seek many sexual encounters. He knows that doing so has a non-insignificant chance of contracting AIDS and hence is welfare-reducing. He has all the relevant feasible information and yet chooses (due to the powerful sex drive) x that he knows to be of lower expected welfare. (This is not really a hypothetical example. I am confident that, out of 100 normal adult males, at least 10 have actually made such choices. If one wants more solid evidence, one may look at the frequency of prostitution and extra-marital sex.) Should we call this preference informed as the person has all the relevant feasible information, or uniformed because it is not in agreement with his real interests?

The above two causes of irrational preference illustrate the point that, due either to imperfection in our endowed faculty or the biological bias in favour of reproductive fitness, we may do things not quite consistent with our welfare. The issue here is that, for normative purposes, should we use welfare or actual preferences/behavior. Clearly, we should use welfare instead of behaviour dictated by biological fitness. An old Chinese dictum says, "Out of the three un-filial acts, not having offspring is the greatest". However, for the human species as a whole, we are certainly not getting smaller in population size. Moreover, a long-run social welfare function accounting for the welfare of future generations should account for that. If we go for biological fitness, we will prefer unlimited procreation even if that means that we will all be suffering as compared to a smaller population with a higher aggregate welfare. 'We' are the feeling selves that care ultimately about our welfare (positive minus negative affective feelings). We are not them, the unfeeling genes that, through random mutation and natural selection, programmed us to maximize fitness. Unlike other species who are almost completely controlled by their genes and the environment, we have learned to change our fate by using such measures as birth controls. For normative issues, it is our welfare, rather than the selected random dictates of the unfeeling genes, that should count. (On a survey of different concepts of individual welfare, see Ackerman et.al 1997; Diener et al. 2018.)

On top of the above two biological causes, there is another source of imperfect rationality. An individual may stick rigidly to some habit, custom, 'principles', or the like even if he knows that this is detrimental to his welfare and the welfare of others even in the long run, taking into account all effects and repercussions. Customs, rules, moral principles, etc. have a rational basis as they may provide simple guides to behaviour which may be, at least on the whole, conducive to social welfare. It would be too cumbersome and time-consuming if an individual were to weigh the gain and loss in terms of social welfare or his own welfare each time he has to make a decision. Thus he may stick to his routine, rules, principles, etc., without thinking about the gain and loss. If this results occasionally in decisions inconsistent with promoting his welfare and the welfare of others, it may be regarded as a cost in pursuing generally good rules. If, say, there is a change in circumstances, the adherence to some rules may result in persistent net losses in welfare, taking everything into account. An individual may stick to these rules without knowing that they are no longer conducive to welfare. Then the divergence between preference and welfare can be traced to ignorance. If he knows this and yet sticks to the rules, he is irrational.

Many readers may disagree with the definition of irrationality adopted here. For example, suppose a man sticks rigidly to the principle of honesty and would not tell a lie even if that would save his life and contribute to the welfare of others, taking everything into account. According to our definition here, he is acting irrationally. To those (like Kant) who are willing to accept honesty as an ultimate good in itself, he may not be irrational. (For our case against Kant's categorical imperatives, see Chap. 5.) But let us consider such questions as: Why shouldn't a person tell a lie? Shouldn't one lie to protect his people from a cruel invading army? If we press hard enough with such questions, I believe that most people would ultimately rely on welfare as the justification for any moral principles such as honesty. Personally, I take the (weighted or unweighted) aggregate welfare of all sentient creatures, or a part thereof, as the only rational ultimate end (my basic value judgment; more in Chap. 5), and hence define irrationality accordingly. I know the controversial nature of this definition. But fortunately, one does not have to agree on the definition of irrationality given here to agree with the arguments presented in this book. If preferred, the word 'irrational' as used here could be taken to read 'irrational according to the objective of welfare maximization'.

However, are moral principles really fundamental? Before the evolution or development of morality and the like, we (perhaps still in the form of apes or even earlier ones) had no moral or other principles, no concept of commitments and justice, etc. Self-interest dominated entirely, although this does not exclude genetically endowed apparent 'altruism' for the maximization of inclusive fitness. As we evolved and increasingly relied on our high intelligence and social interaction for survival, the instinct for moral feelings also evolved which helped our survival by enhancing cooperation. This was enhanced by learning the importance of such moral practices as honesty in improving our struggle against nature (including wild animals) and against competing human groups. No one can deny that the initial evolution/development of morality must be purely instrumental (in enhancing either our welfare or our survival and reproduction fitness) as there existed no morality to begin with. We then learned and taught our children and students to value moral principles; this was first done to increase the degree of adherence to these principles, and consequently, our welfare. Eventually, some, if not most, people came to value these principles in themselves (i.e. regarding them as of intrinsic values) by learning and probably also by instinct. The evolution of such commitment enhancing devices as blushing can be fitness-enhancing; see Frank (1987). Failing to see the ultimate value is a kind of illusion fostered by learning (I dare not say indoctrination) and perhaps genetics. However, I personally have great moral respect for people with such illusions. They most probably make better citizens, friends and colleagues. But illusions they are nevertheless, at least at the ultimate analytical or critical level. While these illusions are on the whole positive (in maintaining moral standards), they do have costs, for example, in delaying the rejection of certain outdated moral principles.

While we recognize the three sources of divergence between welfare and utility discussed above, it is convenient to ignore the divergence except when we come to discuss problems (such as merit goods and the materialistic bias; Ng 2003 and chapters below) where the divergence is important. In other words, in the absence of specific evidence/considerations to the contrary, we assume that, as a rule, each individual is the best judge of her own happiness/welfare and chooses to maximize her welfare. Then the question of happiness/welfare measurability coincides with that of utility measurability, as discussed in Chap. 6.

One real-world example where the violation of the preferences of people actually improved their welfare happened decades ago (in mid 1960s) in Singapore under Lee Kuan Yew's government. Lee decided to expropriate a piece of land used as a cemetery for certain public development without sufficient compensation. Existing tombs there had to be evacuated for reburial elsewhere. Such an excavation is regarded as an extreme disturbance of the peace of the dead and most survived children would not take millions of US dollars to accept such excavations. Even if the government had only to pay a small fraction of the amount people were willing to accept, the public development would certainly have turned out to involve net negative benefits. However, I certainly agree with Mr. Lee that the government should look after the welfare of existing (and future) people rather than that of the dead, even if this has to be in violation of the preferences of the people now. This welfare-improving decision in favour of development would not only certainly fail to pass the traditional cost-benefit test based on preference, it would also likely fail to pass the public choice test of democratic voting (also based on preference).

It is interesting to examine why preference fails in this case. First, it is partly due to the external costs created by the tradition of excessive respect for the 'peace of the dead'. An individual failing to show due respect would run the risk of social disrespect. Some due respect for the dead may serve some useful function but it has become excessive due to a complex process of interaction, including the individually rational but socially harmful strategy of pretending to be very respectful. If this failure can be explained in the traditional analysis in terms of external costs, the next failure cannot. Secondly, even abstracting away the danger of social disrespect, individuals may have genuine preference for showing extremely high respect for the peace of the dead due to cultural influence. They may genuinely feel the importance of avoiding the excavation of the remains of their ancestors. However, if the decision for compulsory acquisition was made by the government, they would accept it as unavoidable and beyond their control and hence would suffer little loss in welfare. It is thus more than a publicness problem. If the decision were put to a vote, most of them may feel compelled by the respect for the dead to vote against excavation and development. However, if the decision were made for them by the government, most of them would not feel too distressed. Thus, Lee's decision almost certainly increased social welfare despite being against the preferences of the people. (However, this example has some degree of exceptionality and does not justify autocratic decisions against the will of people in most cases.)

The Singapore example above is similar to the situation in ancient China (much less so now, but still applicable to some extent). It was a compelling duty of children to give a deceased parent a decent burial. Thus, one often reads in novels or watches in films how a poor man willingly sold himself to become a slave for a few years in order to give his deceased parent a decent burial. If the prevailing law does not allow such servitude, such a person will not become a slave, improving his welfare, if not his preference. If the law allows such a sale, he will feel unease without giving his parent a decent burial; if the law does not allow it, he will regard it as beyond his option and will have to contend with a simple burial, without much misgiving.

An interesting question arises as to the way we should classify the second factor accounting for the divergence between preference and welfare discussed above, according to our tripartite classification (imperfect knowledge, concern for the welfare of others, and imperfect rationality). It may be thought that, provided we include the dead under 'others', it should be classified as a concern for the welfare of others. However, until we have more evidence to convince us otherwise, I think that the dead are not capable of having welfare. Hence, it should be classified as imperfect rationality. According to our definition of rationality, it is not (perfectly) rational to have respect for the dead over and above contribution to the welfare of existing and future sentients, and apart from such concerns as the fear of social ostracization.

As an individual typically cares greatly about her own happiness, an individual's satisfaction with life is highly correlated with her happiness. But, again, as one may also care about one's contribution to others, the two may differ, as further discussed in Chap. 4. Many researchers use subjective well-being (SWB) as encompassing both happiness and life satisfaction (e.g. Adler 2017, p. 119). This is one of the reasons that make them think of happiness as multi-dimensional. Throughout this book, I use SWB or (individual) welfare as synonymous with happiness, and use life satisfaction separately. I believe this is less confusing and more consistent with the meaning of the various terms.

References

ACKERMAN, Frank, et al. (1997). Human well-being and economic goals, *Frontier Issues in Economic Thought, vol. 3*, Washington, D.C.: Island Press.
ADLER, Alejandro, UNANUE, Wenceslao, OSIN, Evgeny, RICARD, Matthieu, ALKIRE, Sabina & SELIGMAN, Martin (2017). Psychological wellbeing. In *Happiness Transforming the Development Landscape*, pp. 118–155), The Centre for Bhutan Studies and GNH.
BENJAMIN, Daniel J., HEFFETZ, Ori, KIMBALL, Miles S. & REES-JONES, Alex (2012). What do you think would make you happier? What do you think you would choose? *American Economic Review*, 102(5): 2083–2110.
BERGSTROM, Theodore C. (1996). Economics in a family way. *Journal of Economic Literature*, 34: 1903–1934.
BERRIDGE, K. C. (1999). Pleasure, pain, desire, and dread hidden core processes of emotion, Ch. 27. In Kahneman D, Diener E, Schwartz N (eds), *Well-Being: The Foundations Of Hedonic Psychology*. Russell Sage Foundation, New York, pp. 525–557.
BOWLES, Samuel (2000). Group conflicts, individual interactions, and the evolution of preferences. In S. Durlouf& P. Young (Eds.), *Social Dynamics*. Cambridge, MA: M.I.T. Press.
BOWLES, Samuel & GINTIS, Herbert (2000). Walrasian economics in retrospect. *Quarterly Journal of Economics*, 115(4): 1411–1439.
BOYD, Robert & RICHERSON, Peter J. (1985). *Culture and The Evolutionary Process*, Chicago: Chicago University Press.
CHARNESS, Gary & RABIN, Matthew (2002).Understanding social preferences with simple tests. *Quarterly Journal of Economics,* 117(3): 817–869.
COHEN, L. Jonathan. (1983). The controversy about irrationality. *Behavioral and Brain Sciences*, 6: 510–517.
CRAWFORD, C. & KREPS, D. L. (1998). *Handbook of Evolutionary Psychology*. Mahwah, N.J.: Lawrence Erlbaum.
DIENER, E., LUCAS, R. E., & OISHI, S. (2018). Advances and open questions in the science of subjective well-being. *Collabra: Psychology*, 4(1), 15. DOI: https://doi.org/10.1525/collab ra.115.
DIENER, Ed & TAY, Louis (2017). A scientific review of the remarkable benefits of happiness for successful and healthy living. In *Happiness Transforming the Development Landscape* (pp.90–117). The Centre for Bhutan Studies and GNH.
EVANS, Jonathan St. B. T., & OVER, David E. (1996). *Rationality and Reasoning*. Hove, England: Psychology Press.
HAMILTON, William D. (1964). The genetical evolution of social behaviour.I and II. *Journal of Theoretical Biology*, 7(1): 1–52.
HARROD, Roy F. (1948), Towards a Dynamic Economics, London: Macmillan.
HOFFMAN, Martin L. (1981). Is altruism part of human nature? *Journal of Personality and Social Psychology*, 40: 121–137.

IGAKI T., ROMANOWICH, P., SAKAGAMI, T. (2019). Experiments in psychology: current issues in irrational choice behavior. In: Kawagoe T. & Takizawa H. (eds) *Diversity of Experimental Methods in Economics.* Springer, Singapore. DOI: https://doi.org/10.1007/978-981-13-6065-7_5

KAHNEMAN, D. & TVERSKY, A. (2013). Prospect theory: An analysis of decision under risk. In *Handbook of the fundamentals of financial decision making: Part I* (pp. 99–127).

MONROE, Kristen (1996). *The Heart of Altruism: Perceptions of a Common Humanity.* Cambridge University Press.

NG, Yew-Kwang (1992). Do individuals optimize in inter-temporal consumption/saving decisions? A liberal method to encourage savings. *J of E. Behavior and Organization*, 17: 101–114.

NG, Yew-Kwang (1995). Towards welfare biology: Evolutionary economics of animal consciousness and suffering. *Biology and Philosophy*, 10(3): 255–285. Retrieved from: http://www.springerlink.com/content/uj81758r187l7777/

NG, Yew-Kwang (1996). Happiness surveys: Some comparability issues and an exploratory survey based on just perceivable increments. *Social Indicators Research*, 38 (1): 1–29.

NG, Yew-Kwang & LIU, Po-Ting (2003). Global environmental protection – solving the international public-good problem by empowering the United Nations through cooperation with WTO. *International Journal of Global Environmental Issues*, 3(4): 409–417.

NICOLOSI G. & MAESTRUTTI M. (2016). Evolutionary perspectives in ethics. In: ten Have H. (eds) *Encyclopedia of Global Bioethics.* Springer, Cham

PIGOU, Arthur C. (1912/1929/1932), *Wealth and Welfare.* Later editions (1920, 1924, 1929, 1932) assume the title *The Economics of Welfare.* London: Macmillan.

RAMSEY F. P. (1928). A mathematical theory of saving. *Journal of Economic*, 38: 543–559.

SOBER, Elliot & WILSON, David S. (1998). *Unto Others: The Evolution and Psychology of Unselfish Behavior.* Cambridge, MA: Harvard University Press.

STEIN, Edward (1996). *Without Good Reason: The Rationality Debate in Philosophy and Cognitive Science,* Oxford: Oxford University Press.

WILSON, Kenneth G. (1975). The renormalization group: Critical phenomena and the Kondo problem. *Reviews of Modern Physics,* 47(4): 773–840.

Open Access This chapter is licensed under the terms of the Creative Commons Attribution 4.0 International License (http://creativecommons.org/licenses/by/4.0/), which permits use, sharing, adaptation, distribution and reproduction in any medium or format, as long as you give appropriate credit to the original author(s) and the source, provide a link to the Creative Commons license and indicate if changes were made.

The images or other third party material in this chapter are included in the chapter's Creative Commons license, unless indicated otherwise in a credit line to the material. If material is not included in the chapter's Creative Commons license and your intended use is not permitted by statutory regulation or exceeds the permitted use, you will need to obtain permission directly from the copyright holder.

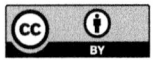

Chapter 3
Some Conceptual Mistakes About Happiness

Abstract Common mistakes regarding happiness such as: happiness cannot be uni-dimensionally measured, happiness is relative, (the concept/nature of) happiness differs over different individuals, happiness cannot be cardinally measured and interpersonally compared (more in Chap. 5), etc. are refuted by considering the evolutionary origin of happiness.

3.1 Why Do We Have Happiness?

Since, by definition, happiness is a subjective affective feeling, one must be conscious to be capable of happiness or unhappiness. A necessary condition for consciousness is being alive. But being alive is not sufficient for being conscious. Living things are defined by the capacity for reproduction. A species may be able to reproduce without the capacity for consciousness.

Consciousness is a principal function of a (sufficiently advanced) brain. For humans, while our brain accounts for about 2–3% of our body weight, it consumes no less than 20% of our total energy consumption (and 85% of that of a sleeping newborn baby). Though many of our brain functions are at the sub-conscious or non-conscious levels, it is clear that consciousness must also be energy-requiring if not more so than our sub/non-conscious functions. We lose consciousness when our brain is not sufficiently supplied with blood. Thus, consciousness must contribute to fitness (for survival and reproduction) and this contribution must more than offset its disproportionate energy requirement for it to survive natural selection (or God's economizing).

How does consciousness contribute to fitness of the organism? It can do so only by affecting its activities. For example, if you are conscious of the imminent attack of a tiger but take no action to run away, such consciousness does not contribute to fitness. But why do we have consciousness that require a lot of energy, and have consciousness that affect activities? Why do we not directly affect the required activities (like running away) without the interim stage of consciousness? These direct actions/reactions are probably true for many lower forms of animals. It is also true for our reflex actions like the arm withdrawal reflex when our fingers are burned. This

© The Author(s) 2022
Y.-K. Ng, *Happiness—Concept, Measurement and Promotion*,
https://doi.org/10.1007/978-981-33-4972-8_3

is the function of our spinal cord. The withdrawal happened before our conscious awareness of the withdrawal. Since actions without the mediation of consciousness are clearly feasible, why do we have consciousness then?

The answer is that for complex enough situations, evolution does not know in advance what actions are good for fitness. For the arm withdrawal reflex, in virtually 99.99% of cases, the best response is to withdraw. Thus, hard-wired arm withdrawal without the mediation of consciousness is best for fitness here. However, the same may not be true for more complex situations. Moreover, the evolution of more species made the environment more complex and hence made simple hard-wired behavioral patterns less fitness appropriate. In a complex situation, the number of all possible combinations of different factors that may affect the appropriate action is astronomical. It thus became too costly to program all the appropriate actions for the huge number of different possible contingencies.

No one knows how consciousness evolved from living things without consciousness. In fact, no one knows how consciousness is possible at all. This hard problem of 'from the material to the mental' is called the world knot and has been debated for more than a thousand years without conclusion. Two and a half decades ago, a well-known philosopher, Dennett (1995) published a book called *Consciousness Explained*. The title was probably made by the publishers instead of the author. I doubt that Dennett himself was arrogant enough to believe that he had consciousness explained. The title is eye-catching. I read and understand the whole book without having consciousness explained to me by even 0.01%! (Not counting our intuitive grasp of what consciousness is without already doing any reading.) Of course, I myself cannot explain it by even 0.000001%.

Once consciousness emerges, it serves the important function of making flexible choices. Instead of just relying on purely hard-wired instincts, on-the-spot decisions after the sizing up of the situation may also play a role. For example, if you see another animal, you may decide whether to 'fight', so that if you win, you get to eat it to enhance your survival; or 'flight' to avoid being eaten up yourself. This increases the fitness of those species capable of such conscious choices, especially when the environments became more complex. However, how did evolution/God ensure that conscious species use their conscious capacity to increase rather than decrease their fitness? This was achieved by endowing the conscious species capable of flexible choices to have affective feelings of happiness and unhappiness, pleasure and pain, or enjoyment and suffering. Activities consistent with survival and reproduction are rewarded with pleasure; opposite activities are penalized with pain. Thus, we find fresh, nutritious food very tasty, especially when we are hungry. The maximization of net happiness (excess of pleasure over pain) then serves as the criterion for a trade-off between different activities and motives, making pleasure the 'common currency' (Cabanac 1992); see also (Broom 2001; Ng 1995) on the evolution of pleasure and pain. From this, we may also infer that dogs, cats, and many other animals (all those capable of making flexible choices) also enjoy eating when hungry. Not only is interpersonal comparison of happiness possible (though with difficulties if precision is required), even interspecies comparison is also possible. (For more details, see Ng 1995, 2015; Carpendale 2015.)

3.1 Why Do We Have Happiness?

On the other hand, the emergence of more species capable of making flexible choices made the environment more complex. This further created a pressure for the evolution of more rational species. This virtuous cycle partly (but still inadequately) explains the fast evolution on Earth to the level of Homo sapiens from non-living things in no more than about 4 billion years (Ng 1996).

My argument more than a quarter century ago, as outlined briefly above, has been supported by recent studies on the emergence of consciousness and affective feelings ('affective neuroscience'), which show that fundamentally similar brain structures support affective reactions in both animals (from amniotes to primates) and humans (e.g. Mashour and Alkire 2013; Blakemore and Vuilleumier 2017). 'There is now abundant experimental evidence indicating that all mammals (possibly many other vertebrates; in fact even invertebrates like crayfish have been found to have worries; see Fossat et al. 2014) have negatively and positively-valenced emotional networks concentrated in homologous brain regions that mediate affective experiences when animals are emotionally aroused. … These brain circuits are situated in homologous subcortical brain regions in all vertebrates tested. Thus, if one activates FEAR arousal circuits in rats, cats or primates, all exhibit similar fear responses' (Panksepp 2011; Abstract; see also Berridge and Kringelbach 2011; Jorge and Vuilleumier 2013; Lewis et al. 2014; Rickard and Vella-Brodrick 2014).

Knowing the evolutionary-biological basis of our capability for happiness helps us to understand happiness issues more deeply and helps us avoid some very common mistakes about happiness, as discussed in the next section.

3.2 Common Mistakes About Happiness

With our concept of happiness or welfare clarified, we now consider some common mistakes. First, many people, including happiness researchers, believe that happiness is multi-dimensional and cannot be reduced to, and measured in a single dimension. It must be conceded that a variety of factors affect happiness; the multi-dimensionality of happiness in this sense is clearly valid. Also, even happy feelings themselves may differ greatly. For one thing, our sense of deliciousness in taste is quite different from our sense of beauty in sight, and similarly for other different senses. Philosophers call them different qualia. The mistake concerns only the point that different happy feelings cannot be reduced into a single dimension to be comparable in terms of total amount, e.g. 'happiness is multi-dimensional and may not be fully assessed by one measure' (Holder and Klassen 2010, p. 426).

The saying 'you cannot compare apples and pears' has of course some validity. For example, you may be able to compare apples and pears in weight, but people care not just about their weights but also their prices, their tastes, their nutritional values, etc. Moreover, different individuals have different preferences in these factors. Thus, in this sense, saying that 'you cannot compare apples and pears' is correct, at least to some extent. However, we must not be absolute in this and regard apples and pears (or some other two items) as totally incomparable. Given a specific aspect of interest, and given sufficient information, we can compare apples and pears. For example, if we just want to compare their relative nutritional values per dollar worth, we can do the comparison if we have enough information about their prices per kg and nutritional values per kg.

Similarly, different happy (and unhappy) feelings may be compared in terms of their significance for total happiness. Our definition of happiness above is one dimensional. For any given interval of time, the (net) happiness of an individual is measured uni-dimensionally by the areas above the line of neutrality minus the areas below that line, as illustrated in Fig. 1 discussed above (Chap. 1). A question arises as to whether an individual really can compare her different affective feelings in a single dimension, such as illustrated in Fig. 1. That an individual must largely be able (but subject to some imperfection as is true for all capabilities) to make such a comparison is ensured by the evolutionary origin of happiness, discussed in the previous section.

An individual in a species capable of flexible choice is often confronted with an either-or choice. If pleasure and pain are to guide fitness maximization, different types of such affective feelings must be capable of being translated into a uni-dimensional scale to allow comparison and choice consistent with fitness maximization. The pleasure of eating and that of having sex may be quite different in qualia, but an individual or a fox has to be able to compare them in a one-dimensional scale to guide the choice between fighting for mating with a female and chasing to eat a chicken. A lexicographical ordering like sex before food will not do. When you are too hungry, you cannot perform in sex! Food before sex will also not do; when you are not too hungry, forgoing a good opportunity to mate may reduce your fitness more than forgoing a meal. As the degree of hungriness varies continuously, you must be able to compare on a one-dimensional scale to choose in a way consistent with fitness maximization. What contributes to fitness (survival and reproduction) more should also yield more happiness to ensure that choices based on welfare maximization by an individual of a rational species are also roughly consistent with fitness maximization (Ng 1995, 2015).

The second common but questionable concept is that 'happiness is relative'. This is correct in some sense as happiness is affected by relative comparison. However, many believe that "the state of 'happiness' [itself] is relative" (Chester 2008), which makes the scientific study of happiness almost impossible, if such beliefs are strictly adhered to. A similarly questionable belief is that happiness and/or 'the concept of happiness differs from person to person' (Guillen-Royo and Velazco 2012, p. 264); see also McGregor and Goldsmith (1998), Uchida (2010).

Consider, 'When younger, happiness stems more from excitement; however, as one gets older, happiness stems more from feeling peaceful' (Mogilner et al. 2011). Moagilner interprets this as evidence for the 'Shifting Meaning of Happiness'. However, it is just that the factors affecting one's happiness may differ for different people with the passage of time and age.

This interesting finding of Mogilner et al. is likely to be universal as well and the reason is likely to be biological. As shown by Ng (1991), due to the cumulative nature of knowledge, it is more important for the young to learn more as their accumulated

3.2 Common Mistakes About Happiness

knowledge is still relatively low and the added knowledge could be used longer; due to the complementarity nature of learning and being adventurous, it is more important for the young to be willing to be adventurous and risk-taking. Thus, we are programmed to derive high happiness from the excitement of taking adventures and risks when young. When we are old, learning is no longer very important; it is then more important to avoid risks and hence, older people derive more happiness from peacefulness.

Even within a species like Homo sapiens, due to differences in individual constitution, experience, culture, education, etc., different individuals may achieve happiness differently and the same factors may affect the happiness of different individuals differently. However, even in this respect, individual differences have been exaggerated. Thus, after reviewing substantial research results, a veteran happiness researcher (Veenhoven 2010a, p. 617) concludes, 'These findings fit the theory that happiness depends very much on the degree to which living conditions fit **universal** human *needs* (liveability theory). They do not fit the theory that happiness depends on culturally variable *wants* (comparison theory) or that happiness is geared by cultural-specific ideas about life (folklore theory).' (Italics original; bold and underline added; see also (Veenhoven 2010b)). Similarly, the finding on the importance of good government for happiness 'is apparently independent of culture' (Ott 2010); the same is true for many other aspects of happiness (e.g. Agbo and Ome 2017).

Another piece of evidence in favour of universality and that cultural differences are not that important is that the many differences between immigrants and local residents are largely reduced, if not eliminated, in just one generation (Yann et al. 2010). Esser (2006, p. 38) concludes that 'the second generation [of immigrants] virtually makes a jump to assimilation … and this finding is stable across all immigrant groups, all cohorts and all periodic fluctuations.' Different but related measures also show similar cross-country similarity (e.g. see Torsheim et al. 2012). It is thus unsurprising that, 'Even if we classify individual affective feelings into different classes such as instinctive, social, and we-world, total happiness may still be represented uni-dimensionally' (Yu and Jiang 2012, p. 977, note 14; 于席正&江莉莉 2012). Also, empirically, 'There is increasing evidence that uni-dimensional well-being models often report comparable and sometimes better fit to multi-dimensional and hierarchical models' (Burns 2020, Abstract).

As different members of the same species, we share many basic biological similarities, including what make us happy and unhappy. Strictly speaking, it is also a mistake (but a lesser one) to say that happiness is relative. Happiness and unhappiness/pain are absolute. However, relative standing, comparisons both to others and to one's own past, and adaptation are very important in affecting happiness, leading people to misleadingly say that 'happiness is relative'. These and other important factors affecting happiness are discussed further in later chapters. Other questionable beliefs such as happiness is not measurable, happiness cannot be cardinally measured, happiness is not interpersonally comparable are discussed in Chap. 6.

References

AGBO, Aaron Adibe & OME, Blessing (2017). Happiness: Meaning and determinants among young adults of the Igbos of Eastern Nigeria. *Journal of Happiness Studies*, 18(1): 151–175.

BERRIDGE, Kent C. & KRINGELBACH, Morten L. (2011). Building a neuroscience of pleasure and well-being. *Theory, Research and Practice*, 1(3).

BLAKEMORE, L. & VUILLEUMIER, P. (2017). An emotional call to action: Integrating affective neuroscience in models of motor control. *Emotion Review*, 9(4).

BROOM, D.M. (2001). Evolution of pain. In D. Morton and L. Soulsby, *Pain: Its Nature and Management in Man and Animals,* Royal Society of Medicine International Congress Symposium Series (pp. 17–25).

BURNS, R. A. (2020). Age-Related Differences in the factor structure of multiple wellbeing indicators in a large multinational European survey. *Journal of Happiness Studies* 21, 37–52. https://doi.org/10.1007/s10902-019-00077-y

CABANAC, Michel (1992). Pleasure: The common currency. *Journal of Theoretical Biology*, 155(2): 173–200.

CARPENDALE, Max (2015). Welfare biology as an extension of biology: Interview with Yew-Kwang Ng, *Relations: Beyond Anthropocentrism*, 3(2): 197–202. Retrived from: http://www.ledonline.it/index.php/Relations/article/view/884

CHESTER, Deborah E. (2008). *Positively Conscious: An Enlightened Look at Life.* AuthorHouse.

DENNETT, Daniel C. (1995). *Conscious Explained.* Penguin.

ESSER, Hartmut (2006). *Migration, Language and Integration.* WZB.

FOSSAT, Pascal, BACQUÉ-CAZENAVE, Julien, DE DEURWAERDÈRE, Philippe, DELBECQUE, Jean-Paul & CATTAERT, Daniel (2014).Anxiety-like behavior in crayfish is controlled by serotonin. *Science*, 344(6189): 1293–1297.

GUILLEN-ROYO, Mònica & VELAZCO, Jackeline (2012). Happy villages and unhappy slums? Understanding happiness determinants in Peru. In H. Selin and G. Davey *Happiness Across Cultures.* Springer Netherlands (pp. 253–70).

HOLDER, Mark & KLASSEN, Andrea (2010). Temperament and happiness in children. *Journal of Happiness Studies*, 11(4): 419–439.

JORGE, Armony & VUILLEUMIER, Patrik (Eds.) (2013).*The Cambridge Handbook of Human Affective Neuroscience.* Cambridge University Press.

LEWIS, Gary J., KANAI, Ryota, REES, Geraint & BATES, Timothy C. (2014). Neural correlates of the 'good life': Eudaimonic well-being is associated with insular cortex volume. *Social Cognitive and Affective Neuroscience*, 9(5): 615–618.

MASHOUR, George A. & ALKIRE, Michael T. (2013). Evolution of consciousness: Phylogeny, ontogeny, and emergence from general anesthesia. *Proceedings of the National Academy of Sciences*, 110(Supplement 2): 10357–10364.

MCGREGOR, Sue L. T. & GOLDSMITH, Elizabeth B. (1998). Expanding our understanding of quality of life, standard of living, and well-being. *Journal of Family and Consumer Sciences*, 90(2): 2–6.

MOGILNER, Cassie, KAMVAR, Sepandar D. & AAKER, Jennifer (2011). The shifting meaning of happiness. *Social Psychological and Personality Science*, 2(4): 395–402.

NG, Yew-Kwang (1991). The paradox of the adventurous young and the cautious old: natural selection vs. rational calculation. *Journal of Theoretical Biology*, 153(3): 339–52.

NG, Yew-Kwang (1995). Towards welfare biology: Evolutionary economics of animal consciousness and suffering. *Biology and Philosophy*, 10(3): 255–285. Retrieved from: http://www.springerlink.com/content/uj81758r18717777/

NG, Yew-Kwang (1996). Happiness surveys: Some comparability issues and an exploratory survey based on just perceivable increments. *Social Indicators Research*, 38 (1): 1–29.

NG, Yew-Kwang (2015). Some conceptual and methodological issues on happiness: Lessons from evolutionary biology. *Singapore Economic Review*, 60(4).

References

OTT, Jan (2010). Happiness, economics and public policy: A critique. *Journal of Happiness Studies*, 11: 125–130.

PANKSEPP, Jaak (2011) Cross-species affective neuroscience decoding of the primal affective experiences of humans and related animals. *PLOS ONE*, 6(9): e21236.

RICKARD, Nikki & VELLA-BRODRICK, Dianne (2014). Changes in well-being: Complementing a psychosocial approach with neurobiological insights. *Social Indicators Research*, 117(2): 437–457.

TORSHEIM, Torbjorn, SAMDAL, Oddrun, RASMUSSEN, Mette, FREEMAN, John, GRIEBLER, Robert & DÜR, Wolfgang (2012). Cross-national measurement invariance of the teacher and classmate support scale. *Social Indicators Research*, 105(1): 145–160.

UCHIDA, Yukiko (2010). A holistic view of happiness: Belief in the negative side of happiness is more prevalent in Japan than in the United States. *Psychologia*, 53(4): 236–245.

VEENHOVEN, Ruut (2010a). Greater happiness for a greater number. *Journal of Happiness Studies*, 11(5): 605–629.

VEENHOVEN, Ruut (2010b). How universal is happiness. In Diener et al. (Eds.) *International Differences in Well-Being* (pp. 328–350).

YANN, Algan, DUSTMANN, Christian, GLITZ, Albrecht & MANNING, Alan (2010). The economic situation of first and second-generation immigrants in France, Germany and the United Kingdom. *Economic Journal*, 120(542): F4–F30.

YU, H.C. & JIANG, L. (2012). A theory of consumption and happiness: The mental-force-field hypothesis. *China Economic Quarterly*, 11(3): 969–996.

于席正, 江莉莉 (2012)。试论消费决策与幸福: 动机—精神力场—行为假说,《经济学 (季刊)》, 11(3):969–96。

Open Access This chapter is licensed under the terms of the Creative Commons Attribution 4.0 International License (http://creativecommons.org/licenses/by/4.0/), which permits use, sharing, adaptation, distribution and reproduction in any medium or format, as long as you give appropriate credit to the original author(s) and the source, provide a link to the Creative Commons license and indicate if changes were made.

The images or other third party material in this chapter are included in the chapter's Creative Commons license, unless indicated otherwise in a credit line to the material. If material is not included in the chapter's Creative Commons license and your intended use is not permitted by statutory regulation or exceeds the permitted use, you will need to obtain permission directly from the copyright holder.

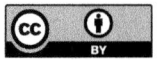

Chapter 4
Happiness or Life Satisfaction?

Abstract Life satisfaction is likely to be more (than happiness) liable to be affected by shifts in the aspiration level, reducing the comparability of the resulting indices. Life satisfaction and/or preference may differ from happiness due to a positive valuation on the contribution to or a concern for the happiness of others. In the presence of such a divergence, levels of life satisfaction may be misleading.

While not denying the usefulness of different concepts like life satisfaction and subjective well-being, this chapter argues that happiness should be preferred in most cases, particularly with respect to what individuals and the society should really be interested in ultimately. Life satisfaction is more liable to a shift in the aspiration level, reducing the comparability of the resulting indices (e.g. Keller 2019). Life satisfaction and/or preference may also differ from happiness due to a concern for the happiness of others. [In the next chapter, a moral philosophical argument in favour of happiness as the only rational ultimate objective is given. All proposed qualifications to this principle can be explained by the effects on the happiness in the future or of others (hence really no qualification) or that their apparent acceptability is due to our imperfect rationality. In Chap. 6, simple ways to improve the accuracy and interpersonal and intertemporal comparability of happiness measurement include using happiness instead of life satisfaction (or other concepts), pinning down the dividing line of the zero amount of net happiness, using an interpersonally valid unit based on the just perceivable increment of happiness, and the complementary use of this method for small samples and the traditional methods for large samples.]

As defined above, our concept of happiness (or SWB or welfare) is subjective ('hedonic' in the philosophical sense), rather than attitudinal, as is the concept of life satisfaction. In other words, it is what one actually *feels* good (and minus the bad feelings to get 'net happiness'), irrespective of what one *regards*. Some authors define happiness or SWB as inclusive of the attitudinal aspect.[1] In my view, it is less

---

[1] For example, Sumner (1996) advance an authentic (informed and autonomous) happiness theory of well-being that has been hotly debated (e.g. Bognar 2010; Tupa 2010; Petersen and Ryberg 2014). Feldman (2004) advances an 'intrinsic attitudinal hedonism' theory of the good life. The intrinsic vs. extrinsic distinction becomes irrelevant if we dispense with the 'attitudinal' requirement and go for happiness in the sense of feeling rather than life satisfaction.

confusing to call such attitudinal concepts of 'happiness' as life satisfaction. Even with the appropriate terminology, there is still the question of which one is more appropriate or important.

We do not have to choose only one of the two and give up the other. Different concepts may serve different purposes and be appropriate or important in different issues. For example, a political party concerned with election victory may be more concerned with people's preference than their welfare, and may thus be more interested in their life satisfaction than their actual feeling of happiness. A statesman or philosopher concerned with people's true welfare may find happiness more relevant than life satisfaction. Also, since we should be concerned with long-term welfare than just the short-term ones, we should also recognize that life satisfaction now may affect happiness in the future. If we abstract from this consideration of effects on future values, or take both concepts (happiness vs. life satisfaction) as both the long-term or a-temporal ones, there are at least two important considerations that make happiness the intrinsically more important concept than life satisfaction. Happiness should be preferred in most cases and particularly with respect to what individuals and the society should really be interested in ultimately. This is related to normative valuation and different persons may have different views. It is difficult if not impossible to have full agreement here. Nevertheless, the views expressed here may be persuasive to some readers. In particular, the two problems of using life satisfaction are discussed in this chapter and the point that it is happiness that is of intrinsic value ultimately is argued in the next chapter.

Since happiness is the ultimate objective in life for most people (and argued to be the only thing of intrinsic value ultimately in the next chapter), life satisfaction is very closely related to happiness. This is supported by the fact that surveys give very similar results whether happiness or life satisfaction is used. However, life satisfaction may yet differ from happiness. Here, we are not concerned with the practical difficulties both from the researcher side and from the side of the subjects in measuring and in forming judgements regarding happiness and life satisfaction, especially the later. It is well-known that such judgments 'are constructions drawn on the spot on the basis of currently available information and circumstances, and thus they are highly unstable and sensitive to changes in the context of inquiry' (Alexandrova 2005, p. 303; also Stundziene 2019). As summarized by Schwarz and Strack (1999), such reports vary with the order of the questions asked, the time of inquiry, the mood of the subject, etc. This unreliability is probably the main reason why Kahneman (1999) prefers the use of 'objective' (a somewhat misleading term since happiness itself is subjective by nature; better understood as 'objectively measured') happiness, measured by the temporal integral of moment-based happiness reports. Here, especially for this and the next paragraphs, the practical problems of reporting and measurement inaccuracy are abstracted away. (For a meta-study of reliability, see Vassar 2008.) Also, Haybron (2007) argue convincingly that 'our attitudes toward our lives can reflect various virtues and vices, such as gratitude, fortitude, ambition, pride, complacency, smugness, softness, low self-regard, etc.' (p.107) and are rather arbitrarily affected by the norm and perspective taken. Even in the absence of these difficulties, happiness and life satisfaction in themselves may still differ.[2]

For simplicity, consider a simply hypothetical example of 1,000 individuals. (Like Einstein's thought experiments, such examples need not be realistic. In fact, deliberate exaggeration from reality is made to drive home the point.) All individuals believe that the only ultimately valuable thing is happiness. However, they are not self-centred and care also for the happiness of other individuals. Thus, they do not just pursue their own happiness but also try to do things that can increase the happiness of others. Evolutionary biology suggests that we are probably so programmed as our sociability is a trait that increases our fitness for survival and reproduction. In fact, even the gene that gives those who possess it a high in helping others has been found; see Bachner-Melman et al., 2005.[3] This, however, does not negate the importance of upbringing and social influences. On some insights on happiness issues from the evolutionary biological perspective, see Ng 2015. Then it is hypothetically possible for the following extreme case (exaggerated to emphasize the point) to happen.

Each individual sacrifices much time, effort, and happiness to do something believed to be good for the society. Due to ignorance, unlucky events, etc., their admirable effort does not pay off. They all end up really unhappy (negative affective feelings more than offset positive ones in aggregate) despite some positive feelings of doing something good for the society. If anyone of them is asked how happy they are, each will say fairly unhappy. However, if asked for life satisfaction, each may say reasonably satisfied, because each believe that what she has done for the society makes her life worthwhile. She is so much satisfied with doing something good for the society that this offsets her own unhappiness. This feeling itself is likely to increase her happiness, but not by enough to make the net happiness positive.

For example, suppose that A, one of these individuals, believes that her good work increases the happiness of each and every other individual by 10 (what unit happiness is measured in is irrelevant to the point being made here; the measurability and interpersonal comparability of happiness are discussed in Chap. 5), giving a total contribution of 9990 to others. This belief increases her net happiness from minus 100 to minus 30. Though she is still unhappy in her own subjective feelings, she thinks that her life is worthy as she has contributed 9990 to the happiness of others. If asked about life satisfaction, she may well say that she is satisfied, though she also says that her happiness is negative. If all the 1,000 individuals are in somewhat similar situations like A, we may get a high degree of life satisfaction and low happiness. Since happiness is really all these individuals ultimately value, the index of life satisfaction may well be misleading in such cases where the two diverge significantly from each other. In this example, the divergence is partly due to the existence of altruism. Other things being equal, the higher the degree of altruism, the larger is the potential divergence between happiness and life satisfaction.

---

[2] Thus our argument here resonates with Haybron's point that 'Life satisfaction in inherently ill-suited to serve as a proxy for well-being' (p. 113). Certain peoples, like the Australian aborigines, may be easier satisfied with life for any given level of happiness; see Biddle (2014).

[3] On the two-way causality of volunteering and happiness, see Lawton et al. (2020).

There is another problem with the concept and measurement of life satisfaction. Though this problem also applies to those of happiness and subjective well-being, the extent of the problem is more serious for life satisfaction. Consider the finding that the average index of life satisfaction for a country such as the U.S. has remained largely unchanged over the last seventy years or so. Can we really be confident that happiness has not increased? Consider a popular method of obtaining the index of life satisfaction. A subject is asked to rate her own index of life satisfaction from the range 0–10, with 0 signifies the least satisfied life and 10 the most satisfied life, taking everything into account. The average index of a country may have remained at say 7. However, it is possible that people fifty years ago were more moderate in their aspiration not only in terms of objective things like income or consumption levels, but also more moderate in terms of subjective happiness. For simplicity, suppose we can use an interpersonal and intertemporal comparable unit of happiness (on which see Chap. 5). Suppose that an average person fifty years ago enjoyed a net happiness level of 700 units and rated herself a life satisfaction index of 7. Now, suppose that an average person enjoys a net happiness level of 1,400 units but still rates herself a life satisfaction index of 7, since her aspired level of happiness is much higher. If so, then an unchanged life satisfaction index may actually hide a doubling in net happiness level. (For some evidence of such a shifting standard and the discussion of related issues, see Hagerty 2003 and Diener and Lucas 2001.)

The above problem may also exist even if the concept of happiness or subjective well-being is used instead, at least for most methods of measurement used currently, including the 0–10 or 0–100 self-anchoring scale. Even if subjects are asked to tick either one of say: very happy, pretty happy, not too happy, and unhappy, the same problem exists. Thus, it may be the case that, people now typically report themselves as 'pretty happy' if their net happiness level is within say the range of 600 to 800 units, while people fifty years ago typically report themselves as 'very happy' for the same range. However, it is likely that, using the concept of life satisfaction makes this problem of changing subjective aspiration more pronounced. This is so because 'satisfaction' is more a concept of relative gratification in relation to the aspiration level. Happiness and subjective well-being are less so, though not completely.

Let me illustrate the point by reporting on the actual situation of a person I know best, myself. For simplicity and to isolate the current issue from the previous issue of the effect of contribution to the happiness of others in affecting one's life satisfaction, let us abstract away any effect on others. If asked to rate my happiness and life satisfaction levels now within the scale of 0–10, I will probably rate both as 9 and tick the box 'very happy'. If I am also asked **now** to rate my happiness and life satisfaction levels **four decades ago**, I will give 6 to happiness level but 8 to life satisfaction. Since I am the same person who experienced my happiness and life satisfaction both now and four decades ago, subject to some imperfection in recollection, I can compare these levels cardinally.[4] (Despite my age, I still have a good memory; I can still recite many poems, some of many hundred words each.) Thus, I can confidently

---

[4] Seidlitz and Diener (1993) found that memory deteriorated **proportionally** for both positive and negative events over a one-year interval. Assuming that this is true for longer period, my current

say that my (net) happiness level now is at least four times that of four decades ago. I may well be inaccurate in my memory but this does not affect the argument here. A change in the correct multiple to 3 or 6 does not change the point to be made. Taking the mid point 5 to be a level of zero net happiness, putting my net happiness level four decades ago as 6 and the current level as 9 provides a roughly correct reflection of the fourfold difference. [$(9-5) = 4\ (6-5)$.] While I am also more satisfied with life now than four decades ago, the increase is certainly much less than doubled, not to mention a three or fourfold increase. This difference between the changes in happiness and in life satisfaction is mainly because four decades ago I was also fairly satisfied; not having experienced a much higher level of happiness, I was fairly satisfied with a net happiness level I now describe as 6. The value of 8 is a good description of my level of life satisfaction then compared to the value of 9 now. But this small increase from 8 to 9 in life satisfaction hides the actual larger than three or fourfold increase in happiness.

Though I now put my net happiness level four decades ago as 6 and my level of life satisfaction then as 8, if I were asked four decades ago for reports on the situation at that time, I would probably have reported 8 for both happiness and life satisfaction. I now describe that lower happiness level as 6 only in comparison to my current much higher happiness level. If we normalize the amount of my (net) happiness four decades ago as 100 (in some subjective unit, not out of 10), my happiness amount now is 400. Suppose my happiness level were to decrease back to 100 five years from now in 2025. If someone asks me in 2025, I will probably report my happiness level as 6 and life satisfaction as also 6. Having experienced the high happiness level at 400, the same level of happiness of 100 that would led me to report a life satisfaction of 8 four decades ago, will in 2025 lead me to report a life satisfaction of only 6. A more important point is this. If my happiness level will be 150 in 2025, I will probably report in 2025 that my happiness level as 6.5 and my life satisfaction level as also 6.5. The crucial comparison now is: Would I prefer:

- X. A life like me four decades ago with a happiness amount of 100 (reported at that time as 8, but reported now as 6) and a life satisfaction of 8; or
- Y. A life like me in 2025 with a happiness amount of 150 (reported as 6.5) and a life satisfaction of 6.5?

It is absolutely clear to me that I will have not the slightest hesitation in choosing Y, due to its 50% higher amount of happiness (150 over the figure of 100 in X), despite its lower figure of life satisfaction (6.5 in Y vs. 8 in X). It is true that, being less satisfied with life in Y than in X should itself reduces the happiness in Y somewhat. However, this effect should have already been taken into account in the happiness figure of 150 that should be inclusive of all affective feelings, including the happy or unhappy feeling in evaluating the life satisfaction. Happiness is the net sum total

---

judgments of past happiness may be quite reliable. See, however, Hagerty (2003) on some difficulties of intertemporal judgments of happiness and life satisfaction.

of all such affective feelings that are valuable to the individual. Thus, the happiness index is more appropriate than the life satisfaction index. (More on this in Chap. 5.)[5]

In the above example concerning myself, the happiness and life satisfaction indices reported contemporarily are the same (8 and 8 four decades ago; 9 and 9 now; etc.). However, cases where the two diverge contemporarily may also be possible. Consider this likely possible though hypothetical example. Consider a fairly happy (amount of happiness = 100) and ambitious young man who reported a happiness level of 7 and life satisfaction of 6 (as his ambition for much higher achievements had far from being realized). Twenty years later, he has experienced much real-life problems and has also come to know many miseries of others, etc. His own happiness amount drops from 100 to 50. He then reports his happiness as 6 but his life satisfaction as 7. His life satisfaction index goes up despite a drop in the actual happiness amount and the reported level because of a much lower level of ambition. The crucial question is: If you have the chance to live only one of these two periods of his life, which one would you want? The earlier one with higher happiness and lower life satisfaction, or the later one with lower happiness but higher life satisfaction? I believe that most people, myself included, will choose the former. The answer to this question largely depends on whether one takes happiness or life satisfaction to be intrinsically valuable, ultimately speaking. The next chapter argues for happiness as the only intrinsic value. Also, by taking psychological happiness in the sense of feeling good instead of life satisfaction or 'attitudinal' happiness as of the ultimate value, many controversies in moral philosophy may be resolved; an example is discussed in Appendix A.

References

ALEXANDROVA, Anna (2005). Subjective well-being and Kahneman's 'objective happiness'. *Journal of Happiness Studies, 6*: 301–324.
BACHNER-MELMAN, R., GRITSENKO, I., NEMANOV, L., ZOHAR, A. H., DINA, C. & EBSTEIN, R. P. (2005). Dopaminergic polymorphisms associated with self-report measures of human altruism: A fresh phenotype for the dopamine D4 receptor. *Molecular Psychiatry, 10*, 333–335.
BIDDLE, Nicholas. (2014). Measuring and analysing the wellbeing of Australia's indigenous population. *Social Indicators Research, 116*(3), 713–729.
BOGNAR, Greg. (2010). Authentic happiness. *Utilitas, 22*(3), 272–284.

---

[5] While recognizing that a host of factors affect life satisfaction, if we abstract away factors like contributions and achievements, and concentrate on factors emphasized in the last three paragraphs, life satisfaction may largely be an increasing function of current happiness, the relative amount of current happiness to the aspiration level, and the change in happiness, i.e. $LS = F(H, H/H^e, \Delta H/H)$, where H^e is the aspiration level of happiness and ΔH is the change in happiness (from the previous level). A specific function is $LS = 5 + \frac{1}{2} \log(H/H^e) \pm \frac{1}{2} \log|\Delta H/H|$, where the figure of 5 is to represent the level of neutrality out of the range 0–10, and the last term on the log of the absolute value of $\Delta H/H$ is to be added if ΔH is positive and to be subtracted if negative. If we operate with figures of H within hundreds or thousands and ratios that are not extreme, this function gives reasonable values within the range 0–10.

References

DIENER, Ed & LUCAS, Richard, E. (2001). Explaining differences in societal levels of happiness: Relative standards, need fulfillment, culture, and evaluation theory. *Journal of Happiness Studies,* 1: 41–78.

FELDMAN, Fred. (2004). *Pleasure and the Good Life.* New York: Oxford University Press.

HAGERTY, Michael R. (2003). Was life better in the "good old days"? Intertemporal judgments of life satisfaction. *Journal of Happiness Studies, 4,* 115–139.

HAYBRON, Daniel M. (2007). Life satisfaction, ethical reflection, and the science of happiness. *Journal of Happiness Studies, 8,* 99–138.

KAHNEMAN, Daniel, DIENER, Ed & SCHWARZ, Norbert, (Ed.). (1999). *Well-Being: The Foundations of Hedonic Psychology.* New York, NY, US: Russell Sage Foundation.

KELLER, Tamás. (2019). Caught in the monkey trap: Elaborating the hypothesis for why income aspiration decreases life satisfaction. *Journal of Happiness Studies, 20*(3), 829–840.

LAWTON, R.N., GRAMATKI, I., WATT, W. et al. (2020). Does Volunteering Make Us Happier, or Are Happier People More Likely to Volunteer? Addressing the Problem of Reverse Causality When Estimating the Wellbeing Impacts of Volunteering. *Journal of Happiness Studies.* DOI: https://doi.org/10.1007/s10902-020-00242-8

NG, Yew-Kwang (2015). Some conceptual and methodological issues on happiness: Lessons from evolutionary biology. *Singapore Economic Review, 60*(4).

PETERSEN, Thomas S. & RYBERG, Jesper. (2014). *Welfare hedonism and authentic happiness* (pp. 7033–7037). In Encyclopaedia of Quality of Life and Well-Being Research: Springer.

SCHWARZ, Norbert & STRACK, Fritz. (1999). Reports of subjective well-being: Judgmental processes and their methodological implications. In D. Kahneman, E. Diener, & N. Schwarz (Eds.), *Well-being: The Foundations of Hedonic Psychology* (pp. 61–84). New York: Russell Sage Foundation.

SEIDLITZ, Larry & DIENER, Ed (1993). Memory for positive versus negative life events: Theories for the differences between happy and unhappy persons. *Journal of Personality and Social Psychology,* 64: 654–664.

STUNDZIENE, Alina. (2019). Human Welfare: Can we trust what they say? *Journal of Happiness Studies, 20*(2), 579–604.

SUMNER, Leonard W. (1996). *Welfare, Happiness and Ethics.* New York: Clarendon Press.

TUPA, Anton. (2010). A critique of Sumner's account of welfare. *Utilitas, 22*(1), 36–51.

VASSAR, Matt. (2008). A note on the score reliability of the satisfaction with life scale: An RG study. *Social Indicators Research, 86,* 47–57.

Open Access This chapter is licensed under the terms of the Creative Commons Attribution 4.0 International License (http://creativecommons.org/licenses/by/4.0/), which permits use, sharing, adaptation, distribution and reproduction in any medium or format, as long as you give appropriate credit to the original author(s) and the source, provide a link to the Creative Commons license and indicate if changes were made.

The images or other third party material in this chapter are included in the chapter's Creative Commons license, unless indicated otherwise in a credit line to the material. If material is not included in the chapter's Creative Commons license and your intended use is not permitted by statutory regulation or exceeds the permitted use, you will need to obtain permission directly from the copyright holder.

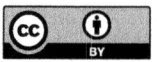

Chapter 5
Happiness as the Only Intrinsic Value

Abstract As happiness is directly experienced by the individual as valuable, its normative value needs no additional justification. Things like institutions and moral principles may be used to promote happiness directly and indirectly. In time, they may be mistakenly valued for their own sake, while ultimately their values should be based on their contribution to happiness. We are born, brought up, and socially influenced to have certain preferences which are largely consistent with our own happiness. Where they diverge, then apart from the effects on the happiness in the future and of others (hence really no divergence in the longer/wider perspective of happiness), ultimately it is happiness that is really consistent with rationality. Arguments for happiness as the only intrinsic value are made and defended against objections or opposite arguments (including 'Rather be unhappy Socrates than a happy pig', Kant's categorical imperatives, Rawls' maximin, etc.). The apparent acceptability of these opposing positions is due either to our imperfect rationality and/or inadequate account on the effects in the future and on others.

Our argument in the previous chapter for preferring happiness when it diverges from life satisfaction is based on the belief that happiness is ultimately speaking, the only thing of intrinsic value. After arguing for this in Sect. 5.1, we also consider some common objections in Sect. 5.2. The non-welfarist position of Kant's categorical imperatives and 'anti-utilitarian' position of Rawls are criticized in Sects. 5.3 and 5.4 respectively. Further objections are discussed in Appendix B.

5.1 Happiness as the Only Intrinsic Value

A number of reasons may make life satisfaction to diverge from happiness. In the previous chapter, we discuss a case where a person A may have low or even negative (net) happiness but yet have high life satisfaction as she believes that she has made significant contributions towards increasing the happiness of others. Whether this belief is correct or not, it can be argued that only her happiness, not her life satisfaction, should be counted in the ultimate social objective. For simplicity, consider only the extreme cases where her belief is either entirely correct or entirely wrong. The intermediate cases are also taken care of by the combination of the arguments for each of the two pure cases.

If A's belief is incorrect, she did not actually contribute to raising the happiness of other individuals. Her belief that she did so may increase her own happiness. If so, that increased happiness is already counted in the social objective that takes account of her happiness. If A's belief is correct, she did contribute to raising the happiness of other individuals. The higher happiness levels of other individuals from her contribution are already counted in a social objective function[1] that takes account of the welfare or happiness levels of all individuals. ('Welfare' and 'happiness' are used interchangeably as a happiness definition of welfare is adopted.)[2] Knowing or believing that her contribution has made other individuals happier probably makes A happier. However, A's happiness level may remain low, though her life satisfaction level may be fairly high. It should be the low happiness level rather than the high life satisfaction level that should count towards social welfare. Why?

Suppose a person B does voluntary social work that contributes to the happiness of say some elderly people. Obviously, the higher happiness levels of these elderly people count towards social welfare. Moreover, if B himself gets happiness from the social work and/or from knowing/believing that he contributed to the happiness of these elderly people, his higher happiness level should also be counted in social welfare. Thus, it is not the fact that the happiness of other individuals that A helps to raise has already been included within social welfare that precludes the counting of the higher life satisfaction of A. It is just that happiness should be counted but life satisfaction (at least the part that is not based on happiness but on say pure contribution to others or what may be called non-affective altruism) not; why?

Happiness, either in the form of pleasure of the flesh like eating delicious food or having sex or in the form of spiritual fulfilment, is what the individual directly enjoys and hence is inherently valuable to herself. Each and every individual wants to have a high level of happiness for its own sake. Happiness is valuable in itself. This is self-evident to anyone. (If fact, this trait of being able to enjoy and suffer is so important for our survival that individuals completely without this capability are extremely rare, if they have ever existed.) Thus, we do not need any philosophical arguments to justify this (that happiness is valuable in itself). However, we do have to justify the point that, ultimately speaking, only happiness is valuable and that all other valuable things derive their values ultimately from their contributions to happiness. This is done below.

---

[1] Any Paretian social welfare (or objective) function is increasing in individual welfare levels. A utilitarian social welfare function sums all individual welfare levels with equal weights.

[2] Welfare has been used in a variety of senses. Here, only the happiness concept of welfare is used. Even for those who regard welfare as happiness, usually welfare is used to denote longer term happiness. However, either holding the time period concerned the same or taking account of relevant effects in the future, we may use welfare and happiness interchangeably, as already remarked in the text earlier.

5.1 Happiness as the Only Intrinsic Value

First, it may be pointed out that arguments on what is good, valuable or ought to be done, etc. belong to the normative sphere.[3] In contrast to the positive sphere where statements/judgments may be either true or false in some objective sense, value judgments can only be persuasive or not. Thus, it is not logically possible for one to *prove* that only happiness is ultimately or intrinsically valuable or to prove the truth of any other value judgment. One could only try to make the arguments persuasive. However, noting that different people have different views on such normative issues, one does not expect complete agreement.

Let us try to see the persuasiveness or even the compellingness of the main point in a number of steps.[4]

Step 1: In an isolated world of no affective sentients, nothing is of any normative significance

Here, an isolated world means a world/universe that is completed isolated from any other existence in the sense not only of having no informational or any other flows between it and others but also of having no any causal connections (including through gravity or any other force) with any other existence. We may conduct our analysis along the line of Einstein's thought experiments; the question of realism is not a relevant issue. One way to imagine this isolated world is to assume that the real world does not exist. That isolated world is the only existence and hence has no informational or any other causal connections with others. If the whole world has no affective sentients from beginning (if there was a beginning) to end (if there will be an end), it seems clear that nothing is of any normative significance. Here, affective sentients are beings that are capable of enjoying happiness and/or suffering pain/unhappiness. Whether that world is getting warmer or colder, more chaotic or more orderly, etc., nothing will be made better off or worse off. It is of no normative significance.

Step 2: Other things being equal, it is undesirable to inflict pain/unhappiness; it is desirable/valuable to have happiness

If pain/unhappiness is inflicted upon some affective sentient beings without anything desirable, either directly or indirectly, it is clearly undesirable. Similarly, if happiness can be enjoyed without causing anything negative directly or indirectly, it is desirable, as the affective sentient beings (like us humans) can testify to that, at least in principle. This does not rule out the possible desirability of pain/unhappiness that leads to more happiness in the future and/or for others and the possible undesirability of happiness that leads to more unhappiness in the future and/or for others.

---

[3] I use the term 'normative' in its wider sense, being in contrast to 'positive' and inclusive of elements of 'evaluative' and 'prescriptive'.

[4] See also Ng (2000b, Sect. 3.3) for the argument that rational individualism implies welfarism.

Step 3: If something is of normative significance, it must ultimately speaking be due to some effects on the enjoyment of happiness or the suffering of pain/unhappiness.

Comparing Steps 1 and 2 above, it can be seen that, if nothing is of any normative significance in a world of no affective sentients, then in a world with normative significance, the normative significance must be due, directly or indirectly, to the affective feelings (happiness and/or unhappiness) of the affective sentients, since this is the only difference between the two cases.

Consider the situation illustrated in Insert 1 where a host of factors may directly or indirectly affect the affective feelings (happiness and pain) of sentients. These factors and doing things that may affect these factors may thus be important or being of normative significance from Step 2 above. However, if the top box (affective feelings) does not exist right from the beginning and to eternity, then we are in the world of Step 1 and nothing is of any normative significance. Thus, in the world where affective feelings exist and something may be of normative significance, the normative significance must be based on or due to, at least ultimately speaking, on the effects on the normatively important affective feelings (top box in Insert 1).

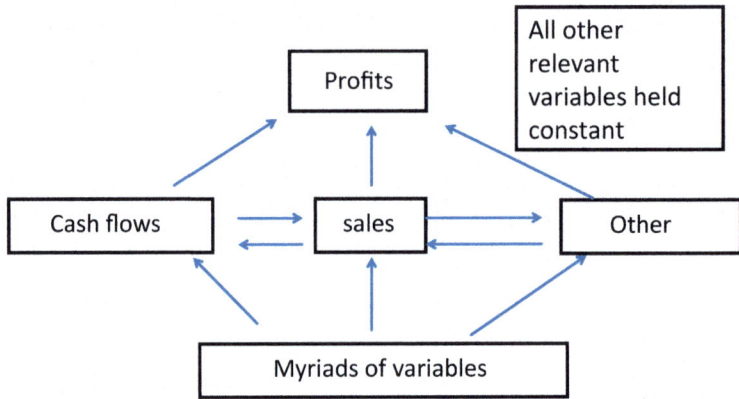

Consider an analogy illustrated in Insert 2 where the final profits of a firm is shown in the top box. The analogy is not perfect because things other than the final profits may be significant, even just to the firm (or its owners). Thus, to make the analogy hold, we have to either assume that things other than profits are not significant, or hold all other things that may be significant unchanged in the comparison, as indicated in the top right box. For example, if the firm is concerned with the welfare of its employees over and above the effects on its final profits, the welfare of its employees must be among those factors that are held unchanged in our comparison. Apart from these factors that are held unchanged, many variables may affect the final profits of the firm directly or indirectly. Assume that, apart from those factors held constant, the firm is only concerned with its final profits and not, say with its cash flows and sales except for their effects on profits. (These effects are usually on the future period. However, to abstract away from the complication of dynamic illustration, we take all the effects as occurring simultaneously or in the a-temporal framework of Insert 2.) Then, any combined changes (e.g. some decrease in cash holding plus some increase in stock holding) that leave the final profits unchanged must be deemed as equally desirable and hence of no evaluative consequences to the firm. Changes that are of consequence must be those that do affect the final profits.

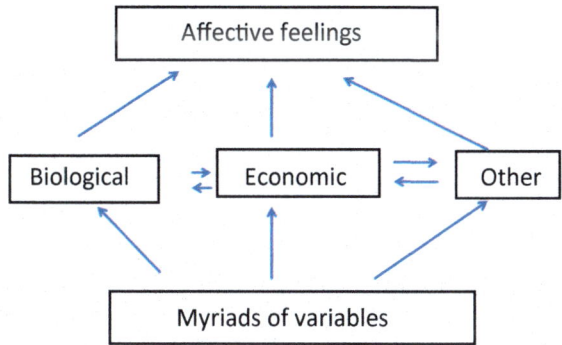

An exogenous change that increases the sales of the firm is usually of positive consequence to the final profits. Thus, some middle managers, especially those in charge of sales, may think it is highly desirable to advertise to increase sales. However, this endogenous increase has significant costs in the form of advertising outlays. The top management should know that even a highly effective advertising may not be desirable if it is too costly. What is desirable or not has to be judged by the net effects on the final profits. Similarly, for the case of Insert 1, what is normatively desirable or not has to be judged by the final effects on affective feelings, ultimately speaking.

Step 4: Something that is not in itself happiness or unhappiness but that may affect happiness or unhappiness either directly or indirectly may also be of normative significance.

If I surreptitiously put a tasteless poison in your coffee, it may have no effect on your enjoyment of that cup of coffee. However, if it makes you seriously sick the next day, it is obviously a bad thing for me to do that, at least if you deserve no punishment and no other benefits comes from this. More indirectly, telling a certain lie may in itself cause no or little unhappiness or may even save some embarrassment, but it may have the indirect undesirable effects of reducing marginally the degree of trust between people and even the degree of observance of other basic moral principles in general, and hence may eventually has more negative effects on happiness and is undesirable as a result.

Step 5: Normative (including moral) principles may be fostered to promote happiness and/or reduce sufferings or to promote things that may be indirectly conducive to happiness.

Due to the reliance of the human species on sociability (including cooperation in hunting) for survival, we have in-born (naturally selected or God-made) abilities like the capability to learn languages, the instinct for moral sentiments and outrages, and even the gene for altruism.[5] However, as the human species also has a long period of childhood for learning, we also rely much on nurture/education, including learning to observe certain principles such as honesty and refraining from littering. This learning takes place at home, in schools, and through social contacts. Most of us benefits greatly from the observance of these principles by most people, largely speaking. Thus, the peer and social pressures against non-observance are big.

Step 6: The adherence of certain outdated normative principles may cause great sufferings.

As circumstances change, certain previously sensible normative principles may no longer be conducive to happiness and may even cause great sufferings. Just a single example suffices to convince. At least in ancient China (for at least a millennium from the Southern Song Dynasty to the recent Qing Dynasty), it was regarded as immoral for a woman to marry twice, even after the early death of her husband (while a man must remarry to have offspring and could even have more than one wives simultaneously). The long tradition to continue adhering to this moral principle cause great sufferings and was the theme of much realistic novels. Very slowly but eventually, this principle was given up over the early decades of the 1900's.

Step 7: Just like people may adhere to inappropriate normative principles, people, including moral philosophers, may inappropriately believe that certain things are valuable independent of and over and above their contributions to happiness.

Influenced both by our inborn inclinations (including moral intuitions for equality and justice) and our upbringings, many people (including learned moral philosophers) may mistakenly believe in the normative significance of things other than happiness and independent of their contributions to happiness. This is a mistake (in the normative sense, being inappropriate, unpersuasive, or even wrong, rather than being false) since it violates Step 3. This may need some elaboration.

Step 3 says that if something is of normative significance, it must ultimately speaking be due to some effects on the enjoyment of happiness or the suffering of pain/unhappiness. These include the effects on future happiness/unhappiness and the effects on the happiness/unhappiness of others, including other individuals and possibly other affective sentients. When we examine closely normative principles/arguments supposedly based on considerations independent of happiness, we can always find that either they are really related, directly or indirectly, to effects on future happiness or effects on the happiness of others, or that the principles are not acceptable.[6]

---

[5] Evolutionary biology suggests that we are probably programmed to be sociable, increasing our fitness for survival and reproduction. In fact, even the gene that gives those who possess it a high in helping others has been found; see Bachner-Melman et al. 2005. This, however, does not negate the importance of upbringing and social influences.

[6] Thus, Mill's distinction of happiness of higher and lower quality is either reducible to quantities of happiness when the indirect effects on others and in the future are taken into account, or not really acceptable.

5.1 Happiness as the Only Intrinsic Value

Our discussion above is analogous to the three levels of 'chan' (禪), a Buddhist teaching on understanding the real world. At the first level, when you see a mountain (or river), it looks like a mountain (river). At the second level, when you see a mountain (river), it does not look like a mountain (river). At the third and highest level, when you see a mountain (river), it still looks like a mountain (river). Here, recognizing the intrinsic importance of happiness is the first level. Recognizing that things other than happiness, like knowledge, freedom, justice, morality, etc. are also important is the second level. Recognizing that why these things are important should ultimately be due to their contributions to happiness is the third and highest level.

It may be thought that what is of ultimate intrinsic values may be multi-factors or multi-dimensional and not just confined to happiness. However, if one (or the society, or any decision maker) has multiple final objectives, one will be in difficulties when these objectives are in conflict with each other. For example, most people including I agree that both freedom of speech and non-racism are good principles that we wish to observe, other things being equal. However, once a radio person made some racist remark and was fired. Here, the two principles are in conflict. Should one always observe one that is ranked higher in importance? How to judge? It is not obvious that non-racism is more important than freedom of speech, or vice versa. My view that these principles are important only because of their contributions to happiness allows us a simple way (in principle, though we may still have difficulties in getting the relevant information) to make decision in the presence of such a conflict of two or more desirable principles. We should roughly estimate the effects on happiness, taking all relevant effects into account. In the example above, perhaps if the remark involves only very slight hint of racism without too much bad effects, perhaps the anchor person should only be warned instead of fired. Whenever we have a conflict of two or more desirable principles/rules, we need some higher criterion to guide our choice. Overall net welfare is the highest criterion that trumps all other principles, as Little puts it (see the interview of Ian Little by Pattanaik and Salles 2005, p. 364, 368).

However, many people have objection to my welfare-supremacy view. To consider all such arguments would require a monograph in itself. Here, let us just consider some examples that can be discussed and answered together in the next Section.[7]

5.2 Answering Some Objections

One is the multi-century old argument that it is better to be the unhappy Socrates than a happy pig. A more modern version of this or a similar argument is the so-called pleasure or experience-machine argument (Nozick 1974); most people prefer their less happy current situations than to be hooked up to pleasure machines that will

---

[7] For these and similar arguments, see, e.g. Elster (1983), Sen (1987), Sumner (1996), Jost and Shiner (2002), Brülde (2007), Chekola (2007). For contrasting views, see Silverstein (2000), Feldman (2004), Tännsjö (2007), Crisp (2006), Haines (2010).

give them much more machine-induced pleasurable feelings. Another argument is on the common dis-preference for happiness based on falsehood. An example is a happy woman whose husband is disloyal to her. These and similar arguments are apparently very persuasive, making modern welfarists and utilitarians largely preference (or attitudinal) utilitarians rather than the classical hedonistic ones. (Welfarism maximizes social welfare as a function only of individual welfare; utilitarianism goes for a social welfare function that is just the unweighted, or equally weighted, sum of individual happiness. Classical utilitarianism maximizes the unweighted sum of individual happiness; preference utilitarianism maximizes the unweighted sum of individual preferences or utilities.) The principle of happiness as the only appropriate ultimate objective is defended below against these arguments.[8]

Consider Mr. C. He believes that, in the presence of uncertainty, the appropriate thing to do is to maximize the expected welfare. (Welfare is used interchangeably with net happiness. For simplicity, consider only choices that do not affect the welfare of others.) Suppose you put C in the privacy of a hotel room with an attractive, young, and willing lady. C can choose to go to bed with her or not to. C knows that the former choice involves a small but not negligible risk of contracting AIDS. He also calculates that the expected welfare of this choice is negative. Nevertheless, he agrees that, provided the lady is beautiful enough and the risk not too high (though high enough to reduce his expected welfare), he will choose to go (or fail to abstain going) to bed with her. This choice of C, though irrational (at least from the welfare point of view), is far from atypical. Rather, I am confident that it applies to at least 80% of adult males, the present writer included. Men are genetically programmed to want to make love to attractive (usually implying healthy) women in their reproductive ages who have not yet conceived (simultaneously explaining why slimness in waist and young girls are attractive), since this helps them to pass on their genes.

After the evolution of consciousness to help making choices (like fight or flight) on the spot by sizing up the situation, evolution (or God) makes sure that consciousness-guided choices are consistent with fitness (for survival and reproduction) by also endowing conscious species with affective feelings. So, activities consistent with fitness (like eating nutritious food when hungry and having sex with reproductive members of the opposite sex) are rewarded with pleasures and fitness-reducing activities (like injuries to the body) are penalized with pain. Thus, fitness-consistent choices are usually also welfare-maximizing choices. However, since the ultimate decisive factor is fitness, the coincidence is not 100% (Ng 1995). In particular, programming the organism to be excessively (from the viewpoint of welfare maximization) in fear of death or to be excessively inclined to mate may be fitness-maximizing. This explains why a man like Mr. C above will likely choose to have sex with the attractive girl even if he knows that this reduces his expected welfare. This example suggests that the choice or preference of a person may not be a perfect guide to what should ultimately be valuable to her.

---

[8] For hedonistic utilitarianism, one needs the additional unweighted sum of utility/happiness part not discussed here. It is argued for in Ng (2000b, Chap. 5).

5.2 Answering Some Objections

Should our ultimate objective be happiness or should it be our preference? Preference may diverge from happiness or welfare for three reasons: a concern for the welfare of others (possibly including animals), ignorance, and irrationality (or imperfect rationality), as discussed in Chap. 10.1007/978-981-33-4972-8_2 above. These three factors are exhaustive as 'irrational preference' is defined to be the preference against one's own welfare due neither to ignorance nor a concern for the welfare of others. Obviously, if the divergence is due to ignorance, happiness should prevail over preference. If due to a concern for the welfare of others, a distinction should be made between the individual and the society. It is admirable for an individual to sacrifice her own happiness for the welfare of others. However, for the society, the social objective should take account of the welfare of all individuals. (For simplicity, we ignore animal welfare here; on which see the final Chap. 10.1007/978-981-33-4972-8_15.) If the divergence is due to irrational preference, it is also clear that happiness should prevail, since preferences based on irrationality are similar to those based on ignorance. For the case of this divergence due to the genetically programmed tendency to mate, it may be pointed out that our (i.e. persons like you and me) welfare is the affective feelings that we enjoy over our life time, not that of our genes that 'aim' at fitness. We should aim at happiness, not fitness. (The maximization of long-term welfare requires sufficiently high fitness though.) We are the feeling persons, not the unfeeling genes. Thus, Mr. C, in his calm and reflective moment, may agree that it is in his interest to resist going to bed with the attractive lady to avoid contracting AIDS. However, due to biology, few men can resist successfully in that hotel room. However, for the ultimate social objective, we should go with his reflective moment rather the moment he was tempted by the attractive lady in the hotel room; we should go with our feeling persons, not with the unfeeling genes.

Just as we are born with the excessive inclination to mate, we are also genetically programmed with certain traits that tend to increase our fitness even if our happiness may be compromised somewhat, perhaps at the margin. One such trait is our inclination to do things rather than just enjoying existing accomplishments or just enjoy the stimulation of a pleasure machine. The drive to achieve helps us to increase our fitness. This drive is also much reinforced by education and social influences. We find such drives so natural and so important that we do not know that, when such drives conflict with our happiness, they (usually only at the margin, as too low a drive level is bad both for fitness and for welfare) are really bad for our true interest, just like the excessive drive to mate in the case of Mr. C in his hotel room. Thus, while it may be true that most persons will reject the pleasure machine option offering many times the amount of happy feelings, the choice of this option (assuming no external costs on others) is the more rational one, just like the choice of not sleeping with the lady.

Will I choose the pleasure machine option? Still not, because I believe that I can contribute to the welfare of others through my work. If I cannot and if hooking up to the machine will not put anyone in misery, I will in fact gladly choose to hook up!⁹ Similarly, I prefer to be a happy pig rather than be a learned philosopher if my philosophy cannot help others, directly or indirectly, to increase happiness by a lot more. My choice may be the exception. However, as explained above, most people (the present author included) are not perfectly rational due to our genetic programs and our upbringings.

We are similarly programmed and socially influenced to be curious and want to find the truth and so on. Thus, our preference for 'authentic happiness' or dispreference for a happy but deluded life may again be explained by either the effects on the happiness in the future or of others, or by our imperfectly rational preferences. For the ultimate social objective, we should go with the rational objective of happiness rather than the imperfectly rational preferences. In fact, it may be argued that it is a mistake for failing to see that happiness is the only rational ultimate objective and all supposed qualifications to this can be explained by the effects on the happiness in the future or of others (hence really no qualification) or that their apparent acceptability is due to our imperfectly rational preferences programmed by our genes and shaped by our upbringings and social interactions. If moral philosophers can see this fundamental point in ethics, they would probably have no difficulties in accepting happiness as the only right ultimate moral principle, making most of the muddled discussion in moral philosophy unnecessary.

This does not deny the value of secondary virtues like truth, autonomy, accomplishment, justice, etc. However, it is important to keep in mind that all these virtues are ultimately based on the effects on happiness. Failure to do so may end up causing great suffering such as the case of blindly adhering to the moral principle of not permitting women to marry twice in ancient China discussed above. Injustice is the denial of due happiness or the undue imposition of unhappiness.¹⁰ Why certain denial is or is not due denial or undue imposition is ultimately also based on the effects on happiness. However, once secondary virtues/principles are accepted, their violation may be detrimental to happiness not only due to the direct effects but also due to indirect effects, including reducing the general adherence to good moral principles and making those believing in the principles concerned less happy. Viewing happiness as ultimately the only thing of value does not preclude taking all these direct and indirect effects into account.

Griffin (2007, p. 147) asks, 'What could be the bridging notion that would allow us to compare a short life of supreme moral achievement with a long ordinary life?' A short life of supreme moral achievement (safeguarding the country in Griffin's example) may be more valuable, but only because it helps others to achieve more happiness, both directly in safeguarding the country and in setting a good example for virtuous and courageous acts. Accepting happiness as the only ultimately valuable

---

⁹ The amount of happiness from the pleasure machine has to be very, very large for it to be worthwhile for all individuals to hook up if that means no further advance in knowledge, science, and technology which may help to increase the happiness of our grandchildren very spectacularly; see Chap. 10.1007/978-981-33-4972-8_12.

¹⁰ Ian Little goes as far as saying not only that happiness is the final criterion but also that happiness or 'welfare can trump justice' (see the interview of Ian Little by Pattanaik and Salles 2005, p. 364, 368).

thing allows us (subject to practical difficulties of estimating the quantitative effects) to compare different secondary values and to make the logical choice when different secondary principles are in conflict.[11]

Most, if not all, objections to happiness as the only ultimate value ignore the effects on others and in the future. For example, consider Hausman's (2010, p. 336) objection: 'A crucial problem with the proposal to diminish the time people spend doing things they find unpleasant is that a myopic policy of maximizing current net pleasure is no more likely to maximize net pleasure over a lifetime than is a policy of maximizing weekly profits likely to maximize profits over a decade.' Obviously, if adequate effects on the future and on others are taken into account, maximizing (net) happiness is not open to such objections.

The above argues in favour of happiness mainly against preference (as the ultimate objective). However, the difference between happiness and life satisfaction and that between happiness and preference are very similar. Thus, our argument in favour of happiness against preference can also be used to argue in favour of happiness against life satisfaction where the two differ.

5.3 Rejecting Kant's Categorical Imperatives

Our welfarist position that ultimately only welfare or happiness is of intrinsic value is different or even inconsistent with some other moral philosophical positions, especially the Kantian. While this is not a place to provide a full refutation of these alternative positions, I will just briefly explain that welfarism/utilitarianism is not inconsistent with the valid parts in Kant (e.g. universalizability; treating humanity not as mere means); and those parts in Kant not consistent with welfarism/utilitarianism are not acceptable (e.g. disclosing the hiding place of potential victims to a murderer). For simplicity, we ignore the difference between utility and welfare discussed in Chap. 2 above.

If you want to quench your thirst, you have to drink something. Drinking something is then a conditional imperative, being conditional on wanting to quench your thirst. A categorical imperative is not conditional on anything; it is something you must do (morally speaking) unconditionally. Accepting some imperatives or moral

---

[11] Our pure happiness theory also avoids many asymmetrical positions difficult to sustain. For example, among others, Brülde (2007) argue against the pure happiness theory based, in my view, either on effects on others or the future or on unacceptable grounds. However, he concludes, 'The pure (unmodified) happiness theory is not a plausible theory of the good life, but it may well be a plausible theory of the bad life" (p. 47). Such asymmetries are difficult to justify. If a happy life may not be good due either to the detrimental effects on others and the future (which I accept as a valid reason but not inconsistent with the pure happiness theory) or to the violation of some principles/virtues not based on happiness (which I reject), then it seems that we should also symmetrically have the result that a miserable life may not be bad due to the favourable effects on the happiness of others and/or the future or due to the observance of some principles/virtues not based on happiness.

principles categorically irrespective of their welfare consequences may certainly be inconsistent with welfarism, as discussed below with reference to Kant.

I have no qualm with Kant's first formulation of universalizability: 'Act only according to that maxim whereby you can at the same time will that it should become a universal law.' (Kant 1785/1993, p. 30; 4:421). Obviously, it is also consistent with welfarism and utilitarianism. Each individual utility or welfare value has the same significance with any anonymous SWF (social welfare function). Since welfarism/utilitarianism does not rule out but rather requires anonymity, there is no inconsistency with universalizability.

Now consider Kant's second formulation of humanity: 'Act in such a way that you treat humanity, whether in your own person or in the person of any other, never merely as a means to an end, but always at the same time as an end' (Kant 1785/1993, p. 36; 4: 429). The consistency of this with welfarism is ambiguous, depending on interpretation.

Kant's imperative of 'no mere means for humanity' may be interpreted in a morally compelling way and as being consistent with welfarism. The central part of treating any person 'never merely as a means to an end, but always at the same time as an end' is certainly consistent with welfarism. Welfarism requires that the utility of each and every individual should enter into the SWF (i.e. is taken into account of) positively. This is inconsistent with treating a person as a mere means, not also as an end. If person is a mere means, his utility does not enter the SWF directly but may only affect social welfare by contributing (as a means) to the utility levels of some other individuals that enter the SWF. Welfarism requires the consideration of the utility of each and every person. We may use a pencil as a mere means. We may also use a person as a means to achieve something, but in doing so, we must also consider her feeling. If we use her as a mere means, not as also an end, then we do not need to consider her feeling, just like we do not have to consider the feeling of a pencil.

In fact, for this compelling part of 'never merely as a means to an end, but always at the same time as an end', I would go beyond humanity and include all sentients capable of welfare (enjoyment and suffering). Animal welfare should be a part of human morality, as discussed in the final Chap. 15.

Both Kant and many interpreters of Kant went beyond the above compelling part of 'not merely a means'. Without entering into a full discussion, I will just mention two points quickly.

First, from his categorical imperative, Kant derived some moral principles too absolutely, to the disregard of possible huge welfare losses. One clearly unacceptable example is Kant's insistence that 'To be truthful (honest) in all declarations is therefore a sacred unconditional command of reason, and not to be limited by any expediency' (Kant 1799; last page), even to an intended murderer about the hiding place of the potential victim. Kant made this clearly absolute imperative in his reply to Benjamin Constant's criticism. Most people, myself clearly included, find this unacceptable.

One reason that led Kant astray is his mistaken all-or-nothing reasoning. This happened in many of his arguments. Just one simple example here. In his argument against stealing, Kant considered the moral proposition that it is permissible to steal.

5.3 Rejecting Kant's Categorical Imperatives

He argued that this proposition would result in a contradiction upon universalization. The concept of stealing itself presupposes the existence of private property rights. However, the universalization of stealing would lead to no property rights, leading to a logical contradiction. This reasoning is based on contrasting only the two opposite extremes of free stealing for all and absolutely no stealing in any circumstances. In the real world, we are always in-between these two non-existent extremes. Most morally upright persons would avoid stealing as far as possible, but may be compelled to steal if that is the only way, say, to avoid starvation of his children to death. Such a morality that allows stealing in some extreme circumstances does not end us up with complete absence of property rights. (For a similar mistake of all-or-nothing comparison by a Nobel laureate ending up with the grave mistake against the sensible taxation of pollution, see Ng 2007.)

Secondly, considering some real-world examples where the observance of some categorical imperatives has ended up in dismal situations may illustrate the unacceptability of sticking to some imperatives without regard to their welfare consequences. As already discussed above, in ancient China, for nearly a thousand years since the Southern Song dynasty in the twelfth century, people virtually universally believed in the categorical imperative that 'one woman should not serve two men/husbands'. This does not just mean that a woman should not marry two husbands at the same time. Rather, it means that, once a woman is married to a man, she should not marry again even after the death of her husband, and even if the death occurs at the wedding night, after the ceremony but before real consummation of the marriage. This imperative or principle was dictated by the sacred unconditional command of chastity, irrespective of its welfare consequences. For many centuries, this imperative led to enormous misery. It was only after many decades of severe criticisms, including by many novelists, that the imperative was gradually given up over the early decades of the twentieth century. The change was partly assisted by the Western thinking of gender equality and women emancipation.

It may be thought that such backward moral principles as 'one woman should not serve two men/husbands' were only observed by ignorant people in a backward country in the past; modern people do not commit such a silly mistake. Actually, right today, almost throughout the whole world and for all countries except one, we have a similar sacrosanct moral principle of categorical imperative that has contributed to unnecessary, intense and prolonged suffering of many people. Those trying to help reduce this suffering have been persecuted and jailed. What is this principle? The sanctity of (human) life.

At least in some important aspects, the belief in the sanctity of life serves some very useful purposes. When a person dies, she can no longer enjoy life. Thus, ending a life prematurely is a grave matter. In addition, living persons are also threatened by this possible premature death. The costs of causing deaths are enormous. Emphasizing the sanctity of life helps to prevent or at least reduce wanton disregard to lives and serves some useful purpose. The mistake consists in absolutising it and divorcing it from welfare. This absolute sanctity leads to the imprisonment of doctors helping desperate patients to end their miserable lives earlier. This has led to much unnecessary suffering.

In conclusion, Kant and other deontic arguments have not refuted welfarism which is consistent with their acceptable parts; those parts inconsistent with welfarism are not really acceptable.

5.4 A Critique of Rawls

If all welfare-independent rights are unacceptable as fundamental moral principles, as argued above, Rawls' (1971) second principle of justice (maximin) is absurd, despite its widespread influence.

Rawls' first principle requires that each person is to have an equal right to the most extensive total system of equal basic liberties compatible with a similar system of liberty for all. I am prepared to accept this first principle on the following understanding:

(1) that it is adopted *because* it promotes the general welfare;
(2) in circumstances where it is disastrous to the general welfare, it may have to be suspended;
(3) in deciding what is the "most extensive total system" and what is compatible ... for all", the ultimate criterion is the general welfare.

A sex maniac may be in favour of freedom to rape and claim that this is compatible with everyone's freedom to rape.[12] It may also happen that the sex maniac is the person of the lowest welfare level such that freedom to rape for all will maximize the welfare of the worst off, hence consistent with the spirit of Rawls' second principle to be discussed below. However, if freedom to rape results in the reduction of the welfare of those raped and scared of being raped by more than (in aggregate) the welfare gains of the rapists (even though the former still have higher welfare levels than the latter group even with freedom to rape), then freedom to rape should be regarded as not compatible with the freedom of not being raped. The "most extensive total system of basic liberties" should then not include the freedom to rape. However, thus interpreted, the first principle is really a device to promote the general welfare. It is not ultimate.

Despite its obvious absurdity, Rawls' second principle is very popular. For example, Temkin believes that, in "one form or another, many philosophers have come to advocate a maximin principle of justice, and one can see why. There is strong appeal to the view that just as it would be right for a mother to devote most of her effort and resources to her neediest child, so it would be right for society to devote most of its effort and resources to its neediest members" (Temkin 1986 p. 109). In my view, the ethical appealingness of this argument as well as that of the maximin principle of justice itself is not difficult to refute.

---

[12] It is true that Rawls would argue that freedom to rape is not a basic liberty while the right to non-violation of body is. However, how do we determine what are basic liberties? Either it is based on the welfarist principle or it is open to the objection of the last subsection on the unacceptability of rights-based ethics.

5.4 A Critique of Rawls

I agree that, in most cases, a mother should devote more, and in many cases, most of her effort and resources to her neediest child, but only because this maximizes the welfare of the whole family (ignoring effects on others for simplicity). The most disadvantaged child is usually the neediest one because he/she will suffer most in the absence of extra help. Also, the extra help for the neediest also promotes the good spirit of helping the needy. Thus, the extra care for the most disadvantaged need not be inconsistent with overall welfare maximization. However, the maximin principle requires the mother to go much further.

For simplicity, suppose that the mother is faced with only two alternatives. One is to go away with the most disadvantaged child to live in a mountain resort for certain marginal benefit to the health of the sick child. The other is to stay at home looking after all the five children but still with possibly more care for the most disadvantaged one. Suppose the two welfare profiles for the children are

$$WP_A = (10, 10, 10, 10, 9)$$
$$WP_H = (9000, 9000, 9000, 9000, 8)$$

and that the mother is indifferent herself and no one else is affected by the choice. The maximin principle requires choosing WP_A. This, in comparison to the alternative of staying at home, increases the welfare of the worst-off child from 8 to 9 at the costs of a huge reduction in welfare (from 9000 to 10) for every other child. No sane mother in the world would make such an absurd choice.

Note that the welfare profiles WP_A and WP_H above are ultimate outcomes, as must be the case for all discussion of the ultimate ethical principles. Thus, the more equal welfare profile of WP_A would not promote further gain in welfare through, say, a more harmonious family relationship. Such effects, if any, should already have been incorporated into WP_A and WP_H.

Consider the much-cherished principle, "From each according to his ability; to each according to his needs" (which I personally approve, assuming no disincentive effect). Why doesn't it read, "An equal amount of work from each; an equal amount of income to each"? If a weak man is tired by four hours of work, it is better for a stronger man to work longer to relieve him. Similarly, if the worst-off child will not gain much more happiness by extra effort and resources, it is better that these resources be spent on other children.

In the original position, behind the veil of ignorance as to which child I would be born into, I would have not the slightest hesitation in wishing my mother to maximize the welfare of all the children, i.e. the unweighted sum of all children's welfare (the welfare of the mother and that of any other person are being held constant in this comparison). This maximizes mine as well as other children's expected welfare.

It is sometimes argued that a risk-averse person may not want to maximize expected welfare. It is quite rational to be risk-averse with respect to income or any other objective rewards since one may have, with good reasons, diminishing marginal utility/welfare of income. But since utility/welfare is the ultimate objective one is presumably maximizing, it is not rational not to maximize expected utility/welfare, if the relevant utility/welfare profiles already included all relevant effects, including such things as anxiety, excitement, etc. which explain most paradoxes of choices involving risk such as the Allais (Allais and Hagen 1979); see Harsanyi (1976, Part A) and Ng (1984). Secondly, if one chooses to be risk-averse with respect to welfare, it is still impossible to reasonably justify an *absolute* degree of risk-averseness as implied by the maximin principle.

After the lifting of the veil of ignorance, I would still think that it is right for my mother or anyone's mother to maximize the welfare of all children together whether I were the worst-off child or not. Again, my bias in favour of my own welfare may mean that I would hope that my mother would spend more effort and resources on *me* somewhat beyond the level justified by unweighted sum maximization. (But I think it is unjust for my mother to follow the partial wish of any child.) However, even then, I would definitely not *want* my mother to maximin in my favour, implying a zero trade-off on the welfares of my brothers and sisters as long as their welfares remain higher than mine. Thus, given the welfare profiles WP_A and WP_H above, even if I were the worst-off child, I would want my mother to choose WP_H. It may be thought that since my welfare is higher in WP_A, I could not have wanted my mother to choose WP_H. This ignores the differences between welfare and preference due to a concern for the welfares of others as discussed in Chap. 2 above.

From the above, it may be concluded that the maximin principle of justice is not only utterly unacceptable but an ethical principle similar to the one in favour of its adoption seems to require *the worst-off group* itself not to accept it. Why then is the principle so popular? One possible explanation is that it appeals to the guilt feeling of the better-off. They have admirable sympathy for the worst-off but yet are not prepared and/or find it ineffective to alleviate this by substantial personal contribution to the worst-off (by charity or the like). Paying lip service by advocating the maximin principle of justice is a much more cost-effective way of alleviating their sense of guilt. Of course, this explanation need not apply to all advocates of maximin.

In addition to those considered in this chapter, other arguments against happiness as the only intrinsic value are discussed in Appendix B.

References

ALLAIS, Maurice. & HAGEN, Ole. (1979). *Expected Utility Hypotheses and the Allais Paradox.* Dordrecht: Reidel Publishing Company.
BACHNER-MELMAN, R., GRITSENKO, I., NEMANOV, L., ZOHAR, A. H., DINA, C. & EBSTEIN, R. P. (2005). Dopaminergic polymorphisms associated with self-report measures of human altruism: A fresh phenotype for the dopamine D4 receptor. *Molecular Psychiatry, 10*, 333–335.
BRÜLDE, Bengt (2007). Happiness and the good life. Introduction and conceptual framework. *Journal of Happiness Studies*, 8(1): 1–14.
CHEKOLA, Mark. (2007). Happiness, rationality, autonomy and the good life. *Journal of Happiness Studies, 8*(1), 51–78.
CRISP, Roger. (2006). Hedonism reconsidered. *Philosophy and Phenomenological Research, 73*(3), 619–645.

References

ELSTER, Jon. (1983). *Sour Grapes*. New York: Cambridge University Press.
FELDMAN, Fred. (2004). *Pleasure and the Good Life*. New York: Oxford University Press.
GRIFFIN, James. (2007). What do happiness studies study? *Journal of Happiness Studies, 8*, 139–148.
HAINES, William A. (2010). Hedonism and the variety of goodness. *Utilitas, 22*(2), 148–170.
HARSANYI, John C. (1976). *Essays on Ethics, Social Behaviour, and Scientific Explanation*. Springer.
HAUSMAN, Daniel M. (2010). Hedonism and welfare economics. *Economics and Philosophy*, 26: 321–344.
JOST, Lawrence & SHINER, Roger A. (Ed.). (2002). *Eudaimonia and Well-being: Ancient and Modern Conceptions*. Edmonton: Academic Printing and Publishing.
KANT, Immanuel (1785/1993). *Grounding for the Metaphysics of Morals*. Translated by Ellington, James W. (3rd ed.). Hackett.
KANT, Immanuel (1799/2012). On the supposed right to lie from benevolent motives, Sophia Omni.
NG, Yew-Kwang. (1984). Expected subjective utility: Is the Neumann-Morgenstern utility the same as the neoclassical's? *Social Choice and Welfare, 1*(3), 177–186.
NG, Yew-Kwang. (2000). *Efficiency, Equality, and Public Policy: With a Case for Higher Public Spending*. Basingstoke, Hampshire: Macmillan.
NG, Yew-Kwang (1995). Towards welfare biology: Evolutionary economics of animal consciousness and suffering. *Biology and Philosophy*, 10(3): 255–285. Retrieved from: http://www.springerlink.com/content/uj81758r18717777/
NG, Yew-Kwang (2007). Eternal Coase and external costs: A case for bilateral taxation and amenity rights. *European Journal of Political Economy*, 23: 641-59.
NOZICK, Robert (1974). *Anarchy, State, and Utopia*. New York: Basic Books.
PATTANAIK, Prasanta K. & SALLES, Maurice (2005). An interview with I.M.D. Little.*Social Choice and Welfare*, 25(2–3): 357–68.
SEN, Amartya. (1987). *On Ethics and Economics*. Oxford: Basil Blackwell.
SILVERSTEIN, Matthew. (2000). In defense of happiness: A response to the experience machine. *Social Theory and Practice, 26*, 279–300.
SUMNER, Leonard W. (1996). *Welfare, Happiness and Ethics*. New York: Clarendon Press.
TÄNNSJÖ, Torbjörn. (2007). Narrow hedonism. *Journal of Happiness Studies, 8*, 79–98.
TEMKIN, Larry S. (1986). Inequality. *Philosophy and Public Affairs*, 15: 99–121.

Open Access This chapter is licensed under the terms of the Creative Commons Attribution 4.0 International License (http://creativecommons.org/licenses/by/4.0/), which permits use, sharing, adaptation, distribution and reproduction in any medium or format, as long as you give appropriate credit to the original author(s) and the source, provide a link to the Creative Commons license and indicate if changes were made.

The images or other third party material in this chapter are included in the chapter's Creative Commons license, unless indicated otherwise in a credit line to the material. If material is not included in the chapter's Creative Commons license and your intended use is not permitted by statutory regulation or exceeds the permitted use, you will need to obtain permission directly from the copyright holder.

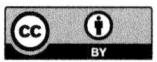

Chapter 6
Happiness Measurability and Interpersonal Comparability

Abstract Simple ways to improve the accuracy and interpersonal and intertemporal comparability of happiness measurement include using happiness instead of life satisfaction (or other concepts), pinning down the dividing line of the zero amount of net happiness, using an interpersonally valid unit based on the just perceivable increment of happiness, and the complementary use of this method for small samples and the traditional methods for large samples.

Economists generally speak in terms of preference or utility. [In modern economics, utility is most commonly used as a representation of preference, in the following sense: $U^i(x) > U^i(y)$ means 'Individual i prefers (alternative/situation/bundle of goods) x to y.] Only since the recent three decades or so that more economists have explicitly studied happiness. However, even if we confine to the older days, utility and happiness did not differ by much. In our definition, they differ only by imperfect information, possible concern for the welfare of others, and irrationality. For most issues concerning individual preference/happiness, especially on traditional economic issues of consumer choice, we typically abstract from imperfect information, irrationality, and pure or non-affective altruism (ruling out a true concern for the welfare of others over and above effects like warm glow). Then, the issues of measurability and interpersonal comparability of either happiness or utility are then essentially similar. In this chapter, we treat them similarly. Section 6.1 argues that happiness (and utility that represents preference) is cardinally measurable and interpersonally comparable, at least in principle. Section 6.2 discusses some ways to improve the accuracy and comparability of happiness in practice. Appendix D also addresses a practical problem in happiness measurement.

6.1 Happiness is Cardinally Measurable and Interpersonally Comparable

I believe that many students of economics, like myself, have at some stage been baffled by the controversies regarding whether happiness or utility is measurable or not measurable, cardinally measurable or just ordinally measurable. Ordinal measurability involves ability to rank. With just ordinal measurability, one can say that utility at x is higher than that at y, but cannot say how many times higher, nor compare differences in utility.

The confusion with respect to utility measurability is partly due to the use of the same term 'utility' both as a measure of subjective satisfaction and as an indicator of objective choice or preference. Another source of confusion is the insufficient distinction between measurability in principle and measurability in practice. For utility as a measure of the subjective satisfaction or happiness of an individual, it seems clear that it is cardinally measurable in principle, though the practical difficulties of such measurements may be very real. These difficulties include inaccuracies and possible insincerity in preference revelation. Moreover, even the individual himself may have difficulties in giving a precise measure. For example, I prefer an apple to an orange and prefer an orange to a pear. If you ask me, 'Do you prefer an apple to an orange more strongly than an orange to a pear? (Question A), then I will say, 'It depends on what kind of fruits I had in the immediate past, what sort of meal I am having'. If all these are known, then I will be able to give a definite answer. Thus, subject to practical difficulties my subjective utility is cardinally measurable. If it was just ordinally measurable, I would not just have some difficulties in answering Question A, I would dismiss it as meaningless. It seems clear that any individual will be able to compare the difference in subjective utility between having an apple and an orange and that between an orange and a house, and able to compare the difference in subjective disutility between a bite of an ant and a sting of a bee and that between a sting of a bee and having his right arm cut off.

It also seems meaningful to say that I was at least twice as happy in 2020 as in 1970. If I have a perfect memory, I may even be able to pin down the ratio of happiness, at say, around 2.8. It also seems sensible for someone to say, 'Had I known the sufferings I had to undergo, I would have committed suicide long ago', or 'If I had to lead such a miserable life, I would wish not to have been born at all!' Hence, it makes sense to speak of negative or positive happiness/utility. Thus, somewhere in the middle, there is something corresponding to zero utility. 'There can be little doubt that an individual, apart from his attitude of preference or indifference to a pair of alternatives, may also desire an alternative not in the sense of preferring it to some other alternative, or may have an aversion towards it not in the sense of contra–preferring it to some other alternative. There seem to be pleasant situations that are intrinsically desirable and painful situations that are intrinsically repugnant. It does not seem unreasonable to postulate that welfare is +ve in the former case and −ve in the latter' (Armstrong 1951, p. 269). This is also effectively the conclusion of Kahneman et al. 1997. Hence it seems clear that utility or welfare as a subjective feeling is in principle measurable in a full cardinal sense.

Economists' Bias Against Utility/Happiness Cardinal Measurability and Interpersonal Comparability

Instead of the subjective sense discussed above, we may use 'utility' purely as an objective indicator of an individual preference ordering and we may not be interested in anything in addition to this ordinal aspect of 'utility'. For example, for certain economic problems like the derivation of demand curves/functions, we only have to assume that a consumer/individual can compare the desirability of different bundles of goods ordinally, i.e. the ability to rank different bundles is sufficient. The same demand function can be derived from the same set of indifference curves with different sets of cardinal utility numbers, provided that the same ranking is preserved. Thus, in this sense, cardinal utility can be assumed away on the ground of Occam's razor for such problems. At least partly due to this, many economists are hostile against cardinal measurability. However, to insist on ordinal utility only (denying the use or cardinal utility) even for other problems, such as happiness studies, social choice[1], optimal population, choices affecting the probabilities of survival (see e.g. Ng 2011, 2016 on the latter issue) where cardinal utilities are needed, is to commit the fallacy of misplaced abstraction. This mistake is similar to insisting that a person must shave off his mustache since that is unnecessary for eating; not allowing for the possibility that he may want to keep his mustache to increase his sex appeal!

The following is representative of the modern textbook hostility against the cardinal measurability and interpersonal comparability of utility. 'There is no way that you or I can measure the amount of utility that a consumer might be able to obtain from a particular good… there can be no accurate scientific assessment of the utility that someone might receive by consuming a frozen dinner or a movie relative to the utility that another person might receive from that same good … Today no one really believes that we can actually measure utils' (Miller 2011, pp. 436–7). There is at least one counter-example to this confident assertion—the present writer.

A probably most widely used textbook in basic economics ('sold millions of copies in more than 40 languages' by 1997) that has lived through 19 editions over 1948-2010 and written by a Nobel laureate puts it bluntly: 'Economists today generally reject the notion of a cardinal, measurable utility' (Samuelson and Nordhaus 2010, p. 89). Note that a cardinal, measurable utility is not just abstracted away as unnecessary, but rejected outright.

Another widely used intermediate microeconomic textbook example on the hostility against cardinal utility: 'But how do we tell if a person likes one bundle twice as much as another? How could you even tell if *you* like one bundle twice as much as another? One could propose various definitions for this kind of assignment: I like one bundle twice as much as another if I am willing to run twice as far to get it, or to wait twice as long, or to gamble for it at twice the odds… Although each of them is a possible interpretation of what it means to want one thing twice as much as

---

[1] The making of social choices involving Pareto non-comparable alternatives, interpersonal comparisons of individual cardinal utilities are needed (Mueller 2003, Chap. 23 and Ng 2000b, Chap. 2).

another, none of them appears to be an especially compelling interpretation' (Varian 2010, pp. 57–8).

Indeed, there is an especially compelling interpretation. Since our ultimate objective is happiness (on which see Chap. 5 above), using the amount of happiness of the individual involved provides a perfect answer to Varian's question, if we ignore the effects on others, which is another issue (slightly touched on above). In addition, the actual amount of happiness enjoyed, but not the amount of utility as representing preference orderings only, could be used to determine well-being even in the presence of preference changes. Thus, using happiness/welfare instead of preference/utility, we may analyze the normative aspects of preference changes.

It is true that the strong and explicit beliefs in the non-cardinal measurability and non-interpersonal comparability of happiness and/or preference (see Chap. 2 on the differences between the two concepts) are held mainly by economists (due to the non-necessity for demand analysis as discussed above). However, even among sociologists and psychologists who study happiness, such beliefs are also very common. For example, sociologist and veteran happiness researcher Veenhoven 'argued that happiness is measured at the ordinal level' (Kalmijn and Veenhoven 2005; Veenhoven 2010, p. 612n). The common belief in the non-cardinality of happiness/utility spans the whole multi-disciplinary happiness studies. Thus, after a cross-disciplinary survey of the issue of cardinality, Kristoffersen (2017, p. 612n) concluded that 'Many scholars (economists and others) are of the opinion that wellbeing data are strictly ordinal in nature, and tend to criticise the common tendency to treat them as cardinal measures'. (See also Kristoffersen 2017.) Levinson (2012, p.873) also mentions that 'economists normally assume utility is ordinal rather than cardinal, and that interpersonal comparisons based on stated happiness are impossible'.

The Compellingness of Cardinal Measurability and Interpersonal Comparability

In fact, the compellingness of the cardinal measurability and interpersonal comparability of happiness/utility is obvious. Consider the following three simple alternatives faced by a person:

A: Her current situation.
B: Her current situation plus being bitten by an ant (non-poisonous one) once.
C: Her current situation plus being thrown bodily into a pool of boiling water

Obviously, she prefers A to B and B to C. If preference/utility is purely ordinal, this is all she can say. However, even you, not being her, know that the intensity of her preference of B over C is at least many thousand times larger than that of A over B. Moreover, you may also be confident that the intensity of her preference of B over C is at least many thousand times larger than that of *your* preference of A over B (interpreting A and B as applied to you).

True, this is interpersonal comparison of utility regarded by Robbins (1932, 1938) as unscientific. In fact, this comparison is solidly based on evolutionary biology, as touched on earlier and also discussed in Appendix C. An ant bite reduces her (and most individuals') fitness by a very small amount and hence induces only a small amount of pain. Being thrown bodily into boiling water threatens ones' survival and must cause great pain and intense attempt to avoid it. Though there may be some degree of interpersonal differences, these are almost certainly less significant than the huge survival difference between an ant bite and being thrown into boiling water. Thus, our degree of confidence in the truth of the comparison above is no less than 99.99%, a degree of certainty envied by all empirical scientists, economists included.

Most people now know that our brain consists of two hemispheres, with the left brain controlling the right side of the body and vice versa. We do not feel this duality as our two brain hemispheres are connected by corpus callosum, making our subjective consciousness unified. However, some patients with serious epilepsy have their two brain hemispheres separated by cutting the connection (to reduce brain interaction). They then behave as if having two centres of consciousness or mind, with their left brain (normally controlling speech) not knowing what their right brain has seen with the left eye, if a blinder is also placed between their two eyes (Gazzaniga, 1970).[2] Thus, two separate brain hemispheres each with independent consciousness may be unified with connection through the corpus callosum. Similarly, if our technology is advanced enough to imitate the connection through the corpus callosum, we could so connect her brain with yours. Then, she could feel your taste of ice cream and you could feel her taste of blueberries. Interpersonal comparison would become almost perfect!

While happiness is cardinally measurable and interpersonally comparable in principle, it is true that the commonly used methods of happiness measurement are not very cardinal and interpersonally very difficult to compare, as mentioned above. The lack in comparability in existing happiness measures makes happiness studies vulnerable to the criticism of doubters of happiness results such as Johns et al. (2007) and Ott (2010). If happiness measures could be based on more comparable methods of measurement, as discussed below, the critics may have less gun powder to use.

6.2 How Could the Measurement of Happiness be Improved?

One reason most economists are skeptical of happiness measurement is that professionally they trust what people do rather than what their say ('cheap talk'). If an individual is willing to pay from her own pocket to actually buy a certain item, economists are willing to accept that she values that item at least at the price paid. If she just says that she values certain thing at a certain value, economists are generally skeptical. Since most if not all existing measurements of happiness are based on how happy people say they are in questionnaire surveys, economists are thus skeptical of their reliability. This skepticism has some validity.

---

[2] However, see Pinto et al. (2017) on the point that, 'although the two hemispheres are completely insulated from each other, the brain as a whole is still able to produce only one conscious agent'.

However, there are persuasive arguments that existing measures, though imperfect, are rather reliable. For example, different measures of happiness correlate well with one another (Fordyce 1988), with recalls of positive versus negative life events (Seidlitz et al. 1997), with reports of friends and family members (Costa and McCrae 1988; Diener 1984; Sandvik et al. 1993, 2009), with physical measures like heart rate and blood pressure measures (Shedler et al. 1993), with EEG measures of prefrontal brain activity (Sutton and Davidson 1997), and with more objective measures of well-being like incidence of depression, poor appetite and sleep (Luttmer 2005). Pavot et al. (1991) finds that respondents reporting that they are very happy tend to smile more. MacCulloch and Di Tella (2000) note that psychologists who study and give advice on happiness for a living use happiness data. 'Presumably, if markets work and there was a better way to study well-being, people who insist on using bad data would be driven out of the market' (pp. 7–8). Moreover, correlations of happiness show remarkably consistency across countries, including developing and transitional (Graham and Pettinato 2001, 2002; Namazie and Sanfey 2001). Dominitz and Manski (1999) examine the scientific basis underlying economists' hostility against subjective data and found it to be 'meager' and 'unfounded'. Rather, 'survey respondents do provide coherent, useful information when queried systematically'; see Manski 2000, p. 132.) Despite remaining problems of happiness measurement (see, e.g. Schwarz and Stracek 1999; Bertrand and Mullainathan 2001), reported happiness indices may be used as good approximations (Frey and Stutzer 2002b; Oishi 2019) and 'happiness surveys are capturing something meaningful about true utility' (Di Tella and MacCulloch 2006, p. 28).

For those economists who are still skeptical or even look down upon and deride at the happiness measures (which actually happened), I call upon them to look at their own backyard. Consider the most important economic variable GDP or GNP. Its measurement is subject to all sorts of inaccuracies, as is well-known to all economists. We used the imperfect measure for many decades. Then came the PPP (purchasing power parity) adjustment which overnight increased the Chinese GDP by 4 times and the Indian GDP by 6 times from this single adjustment alone! Most happiness measures may not be very accurate but I doubt that a 4-times adjustment will ever be necessary for the average figure of any nation.

There are a number of methods to improve the measurement of happiness to increase its accuracy and comparability, including interpersonal and intertemporal comparability. Some of these methods are easier to implement than others. Let us start from the easier ones first.

First, as discussed in the previous chapters, as a rule, using the concept of happiness instead of other concepts like life satisfaction is likely to yield a better result. This is easily implemented.

Secondly, asking subjects to tick from: very happy, pretty happy, not too happy, and unhappy gives very vague results. This is so because phrase like 'not too happy' is vague as to the amount of happiness it represents. It may either represent a positive amount of (net) happiness or a negative amount. Before we use some interpersonal comparable units of happiness measurement (which is more complex, as discussed below), it is difficult to get happiness results that are valid across persons. Different

6.2 How Could the Measurement of Happiness be Improved?

persons may use the same phrase such as 'very happy' to describe different amounts of happiness, and use different phrases to describe the same amount of happiness, making interpersonal comparison difficult. However, there is a well-defined level of happiness that has interpersonal significance. This is the level of zero (net) happiness, or where the amount of positive happiness is just offset by the negative amount of happiness or the amount of unhappiness (pain and sufferings). In terms of Figure 1 above (Chap. 1), it is the case where the area above the line of neutrality equals that below this line. If the net amount of happiness is zero, the value of life to that person herself (i.e. ignoring any effects on others) is neutral. This has an interpersonal significance. A person may have a large amount of positive happiness and also a large amount of unhappiness. Another person may have a small amount of positive happiness and also a small amount of unhappiness. It may be difficult to compare the amount of happiness (or unhappiness) of the first person with that of the second. However, if the amount of positive happiness of each of these two persons just offsets the amount of unhappiness, the net amounts of happiness of both persons are the same, being both equal to zero. Thus, happiness studies should aim to discover, among others, information regarding the proportions of people with happiness levels above, at and below this level of neutrality. This is an interpersonally, intertemporally, internationally, and interculturally comparable and useful piece of information.

When a subject is asked to rate her own happiness within the scale of say 0-10, it is true that most people may use the mid point of 5 to stand for the point of neutrality. However, this is by no means certain or universal. This is particularly so as many Western countries use 50 (out of 100) as the passing mark in exam grading, while the corresponding passing mark is 60 in China. Thus, a brief instruction asking the subject to use 5 to stand for neutrality will increase the informational content of the survey results especially with respect to the comparability of the proportion of people above the neutrality point.

The above improvement can be easily implemented. However, while achieving a significant improvement easily, it does not solve most of the problems of comparability. Society A may have 90% of people above the line of neutrality while society B only has 85%. However, society B may still be a happier one if many of those above neutrality have much higher happiness than society A and most of those below neutrality in society B are only marginally below while most of those below neutrality in society A are significantly below.

To overcome such difficulty of incomparability, I develop (Ng 1996) a method that yields happiness measures that are comparable interpersonally, inter-temporally, and interculturally. It is based on Edgeworth's concept of a just perceptible increment of happiness, but developed to be operational and actually used to conduct an actual survey/measurement.[3] For example, if you prefer two spoons of sugar in a given cup of coffee to 1.5 spoons, you may not know the difference between 2 and 1.99 spoons.

---

[3] The concept of using the faintest unit of pleasure as the unit of measurement may be traced back to Bentham; see Tännsjö (1998).

There exists a difference that makes one just perceivably taste better than the other.[4] Edgeworth took it as axiomatic, or, in his words 'a first principle incapable of proof', that the 'minimum sensible or the just perceivable increments of pleasures for all persons, are equatable (Edgeworth 1881, pp. 7ff., pp. 60 ff.). I (Ng 1975) derived this result as well as the utilitarian social welfare function (SWF), that social welfare is the unweighted sum of individual utilities/welfares, from more basic axioms.

The main axiom is the **Weak Majority Preference Criterion (WMP):** *For any two alternatives x and y, if no individual prefers y to x, and (1) if I, the number of individuals, is even, at least I/2 individuals prefer x to y; (2) if I is odd, at least (I–1)/2 individuals prefer x to y and at least another individual's utility level is not lower in x than in y, then social welfare is higher in x than in y.*

The reason why WMP leads us to the utilitarian SWF is not difficult to see. The criterion WMP requires that individual utility/welfare differences sufficient to give rise to preferences of half of the population must be regarded as socially more significant than utility differences not sufficient to give rise to preferences (or dis-preferences) of another half. Since any group of individuals comprising 50 per cent of the population is an acceptable half, this effectively makes a just–perceivable increment of utility/welfare of any individual an interpersonally comparable unit.[5] (Ignoring the difference between individual preferences and welfare, utility and welfare may be used interchangeably. Where they differ, welfare or happiness should be used, as argued in above; WMP should then be revised to refer to happiness.) The compellingness of this argument is further expounded in Ng & Singer (1981).

Thus, measures of happiness based on the concept just perceivable increment of happiness is not only cardinal but also interpersonally comparable. If we use the same number say one to measure the happiness difference of a just perceivable increment[6] for all individuals, the happiness indices so constructed are interpersonally comparable since each just perceivable increment of happiness is equitable across individuals. Though such measures are more difficult to obtain[7], some such measures may be obtained for some small but representative samples and the results compared with the existing measures taken on larger samples. If some reliable correspondences between the two sets of measures could be established, we may not have to use the more complicated method for the majority of subjects surveyed. The combined use of these two methods may be a good way to tackle the problems of reliability and comparability.

---

[4] Where the time dimension is considered, we may have to use a just perceivable increment over a just perceivable unit of time. Also, given perfect divisibility and continuity in preference, we may have to use a just (maximally) non-perceivable indifference instead of a just perceivable preference.

[5] Given continuity, if we do not equate a just–perceptible increment of utility/welfare of any individual with that of any other individual, then we count the perceptible increment of one person as less important than the imperceptible increment of another and this violates WMP and is also clearly unacceptable.

[6] Or rather, a just unperceivable indifference.

[7] See Argenziano and Gilboa (2019) on some issue of data availability.

The study of happiness is still a very new science. Thus, it has much scope to be improved to increase the accuracy and comparability of happiness measures not only by taking account of the above but also many other issues. Given time and more studies, significant improvements may be expected.

Concluding Summary

Simple ways to improve the accuracy and interpersonal and intertemporal comparability of happiness measurement include using happiness instead of life satisfaction (or other concepts), pinning down the dividing line of the zero amount of net happiness, using an interpersonally valid unit based on the just perceivable increment of happiness, and the complementary use of this method for small samples and the traditional methods for large samples.

References

ARGENZIANO, Rossella & GILBOA, Itzhak (2019). Perception-theoretic foundations of weighted Utilitarianism. *The Economic Journal*, 129 (May), 1511–1528 https://doi.org/10.1111/ecoj.12622.

ARMSTRONG, W. E. (1951). Utility and the theory of welfare. *Oxford Economic Papers, 3*, 257–271.

BERTRAND, Marianne & MULLAINATHAN, Sendhil (2001). Do people mean what they say? Implications for subjective survey data. *American Economic Review*, 91(2): 67-72.

COSTA, P. T., & McCRAE, R. R. (1988). Personality in adulthood: A six-year longitudinal study of self-reports and spouse ratings on the NEO personality inventory. *Journal of Personality and Social Psychology, 54*(5), 853–863.

DIENER, Ed, (1984). Subjective well-being. *Psychological Bulletin*, 95: 542-75.

DI TELLA, Rafael & MACCULLOCH, Robert (2006). Some uses of happiness data in economics. *Journal of Economic Perspectives*, 20(1): 25-46.

DOMINITZ, Jeff & MANSKI, Charles F. (1999). The several cultures of research on subjective expectations. In James P. SMITH & Robert J. WILLIS (Eds.). *Wealth, Work, and Health: Innovations in Measurement in the Social Sciences: Essays in Honor of F. Thomas Juster*. Ann Arbor: University of Michigan Press.

EDGEWORTH, Francis Y. (1881). *Mathematical Psychics: An Essay on the Application of Mathematics to the Moral Sciences*. London: Kegan Paul.

FORDYCE, Michael (1988). A review of research on happiness measures: a sixty second index of happiness and mental health. *Social Indicators Research*, 20: 355-81.

FREY, Bruno S. & STUTZER, Alois (2002). What can economists learn from happiness research? *Journal of Economic Literature*, 40: 402-35.

GAZZANIGA, Michael S. (1970). *The Bisected Brain*. New York: Appleton-Century-Crofts.

GRAHAM, Carol & PETTINATO, Stefano (2001). Happiness, markets, and democracy: Latin America in comparative perspective. *Journal of Happiness Studies, 2*:237–68.

GRAHAM, Carol & PETTINATO, Stefano (2002). Frustrated achievers: Winners, losers, and subjective well being in new market economies. *Journal of Development Studies*, 38(4): 100–140.

JOHNS, Helen & ORMEROD, Paul (2007). Review article on "Happiness, Economics and Public Policy". London: The Institute of Economic Affairs.

KAHNEMAN, Daniel, WAKKER, Peter P. & SARIN, Rakesh (1997). Back to bentham? Explorations of experienced utility. *Quarterly Journal of Economics*, 112(2): 375-405.

KALMIJN, Wim & VEENHOVEN, Ruut (2005). Measuring inequality of happiness in nations: In search for proper statistics. *Journal of Happiness Studies*, 6(4): 357–396.
KRISTOFFERSEN, Ingebjørg (2017). The metrics of subjective wellbeing data: An empirical evaluation of the ordinal and cardinal comparability of life satisfaction scores. *Social Indicators Research*, 130(2): 845–865.
LEVINSON, Arik (2012). Valuing public goods using happiness data: The case of air quality. *Journal of Public Economics*, 96: 869-880.
LUTTMER, Erzo F. (2005). Neighbors as negatives: Relative earnings and well-being. *Quarterly Journal of Economics*, 120(3): 963–1002.
MacCULLOCH, Robert and DI TELLA, Rafael (2000). Partisan social happiness. Harvard Business School Working Paper Series 2000. Available at SSRN: https://ssrn.com/abstract=267362 or http://dx.doi.org/10.2139/ssrn.267362.
MANSKI, Charles F. (2000). Economic analysis of social interactions. *Journal of Economic Perspectives*, 14(3): 115-136.
MILLER, Roger L. (2011). Economics Today. 16th edition. Pearson.
MUELLER, Dennis C. (2003). *Public Choice III.* Cambridge England & New York: Cambridge University Press.
NAMAZIE, Ceema & SANFEY, Peter (2001). Happiness and transition: The case of Kyrgyzstan. *Review of Development Economics*, 5(3): 392-405.
NG, Yew-Kwang (1975). Bentham or Bergson? Finite sensibility, utility functions, and.
NG, Yew-Kwang (1996). Complex niches favour rational species. *Journal of Theoretical Biology*, 179: 303-311.
NG, Yew-Kwang (2000). *Efficiency, Equality, and Public Policy: With a Case for Higher Public Spending.* Basingstoke, Hampshire: Macmillan.
NG, Yew-Kwang (2011). Consumption tradeoff vs. catastrophes avoidance: Implications of some recent results in happiness studies on the economics of climate change, *Climatic Change*,105(1): 109-127,
NG, Yew-Kwang (2016). How welfare biology and commonsense may help to reduce animal suffering, *Animal Sentience*, 2016.007. Target article for peer commentary. http://animalstudiesrepository.org/animsent/vol1/iss7/1/.
NG, Yew-Kwang & SINGER, Peter (1981).An argument for utilitarianism.*Canadian Journal of Philosophy*, 11: 229–239.
OISHI, Shige (2019). Reevaluating the strengths and weaknesses of self-report measures of subjective well-being. https://www.semanticscholar.org/paper/Reevaluating-the-Strengths-and-Weaknesses-of-Self-Oishi/0d063b91daf0bc252b318372200a3aba72fc298a.
OTT, Jan (2010). Greater happiness for a greater number: Some non-controversial options for governments. *Journal of Happiness Studies*, 11(5): 631–47.
PAVOT, William, DIENER, Ed, COLVIN, C. Randall & SANDVIK, Ed (1991). Further validation of the satisfaction with life scale: Evidence for the convergence of well-being measures. *Journal of Personality Assessment*, 57: 149-161.
PINTO, Yair, NEVILLE, David A., OTTEN, Marte, CORBALLIS, Paul M, LAMME, Victor A.F., de HAAN, Edward H.F., FOSCHI, Nicoletta, FABRI, Mara (2017). Split brain: divided perception but undivided consciousness. *Brain*, 140: 1231-7. DOI: https://doi.org/10.1093/brain/aww358.
ROBBINS, Lionel (1932). *An Essay on the Nature and Significance of Economic Science,* London, Macmillan.
ROBBINS, Lionel (1938). Interpersonal comparison of utility: a comment. *Economic Journal*, 48: 635–41.
SAMUELSON, Paul A. and NORDHAUS, William D. (2010). Economics, 19th edition, McGraw-Hill/Irwin.
SANDVIK, Ed, DIENER, Ed & SEIDLITZ, Larry (1993). Subjective well-being: The convergence and stability of self-report and non-self report measures. *Journal of Personality*, 61(3): 317-42.
SANDVIK, Ed, DIENER, Ed & SEIDLITZ, Larry (2009). Subjective well-being: The convergence and stability of self-report and non-self-report measures. In: Diener E. (eds) Assessing

References

Well-Being. Social Indicators Research Series, vol 39. Springer, Dordrecht. DOI: https://doi.org/10.1007/978-90-481-2354-4_6. https://link.springer.com/chapter/10.1007/978-90-481-2354-4_6#citeas.

SCHWARZ, Norbert & STRACK, Fritz (1999). Reports of subjective well-being: Judgmental processes and their methodological implications. In D. Kahneman, E. Diener, & N. Schwarz (Eds.), *Well-being: The Foundations of Hedonic Psychology* (pp. 61-84). New York: Russell Sage Foundation.

SEIDLITZ, Larry, WYER, Robert S. Jr. & DIENER, Ed (1997). Cognitive correlates of subjective well-being: the processing of valenced life events by happy and unhappy persons. *Journal of Research in Personality*, 31(2): 240-56.

SHEDLER, Joanthan, MAYMAN, Martin & MANIS, Melvin. (1993). The illusion of mental health. *American Psychologist*, 48(11): 1117–31.

SUTTON, Steven K. & DAVIDSON, Richard J. (1997). Prefrontal brain symmetry: a biological substrate of the behavioral approach and inhibition systems. *Psychological Science,* 8(3), 204–210.

TÄNNSJÖ, Torbjörn (1998). *Hedonistic Utilitarianism.* Edinburgh: Edinburgh University Press/Columbia University Press.

VARIAN, Hal R. (2010). *Intermediate Microeconomics.* W. W. Norton, 8th International student edition.

Open Access This chapter is licensed under the terms of the Creative Commons Attribution 4.0 International License (http://creativecommons.org/licenses/by/4.0/), which permits use, sharing, adaptation, distribution and reproduction in any medium or format, as long as you give appropriate credit to the original author(s) and the source, provide a link to the Creative Commons license and indicate if changes were made.

The images or other third party material in this chapter are included in the chapter's Creative Commons license, unless indicated otherwise in a credit line to the material. If material is not included in the chapter's Creative Commons license and your intended use is not permitted by statutory regulation or exceeds the permitted use, you will need to obtain permission directly from the copyright holder.

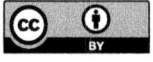

Chapter 7
Does Money Buy Happiness?

Abstract After a relatively low level of survival and comfort, additional consumption does not increase happiness significantly, especially at the social level. At the individual level, people want more due to the relative competition effect which cancels out at the social level. In addition, the adaptation effects and environmental disruption effects also work to limit the contributions of higher consumption and enlarge the gap between expectation and actuality.

Studies by psychologists and sociologists show that, both within a country and across nations, the happiness level of people increases with the income level, but only slightly. For example, using regional and cultural classifications, the Northern European countries with high incomes score top on happiness, followed by the group of English-speaking US, UK, Australia, and Ireland. Central and South-American countries including Brazil come next, followed by the Middle East, the Central European, Southern and Eastern European (Greece, Russia, Turkey, and Yugoslavia), the Indian Sub-continent, and Africa which does not, however, come last. Southern and Western European (France, Italy, and Spain) score significantly lower than Africa. And the last group is East Asia, including the country that leads in income, Japan. Singapore had an income level (per capita) 82.4 times that of India. Even in terms of purchasing power parity instead of using exchange rate, Singapore was still 16.4 time higher than India in income. However, the happiness scores of both countries were exactly the same, both significantly higher than that of Japan. (See Cummins 1998. Cf. Diener and Suh 1999; Inglehart et al. 1998, Table V18. On the East-Asian happiness gap, see Chap. 13). While there are notable cases like Japan and France that are far off the regression line, a statistically significant positive relationship between happiness and income exists cross-nationally. However, over around US$5,000 per capita annually, the correlation disappears (Veenhoven and Timmermans 1998, Fig. 2). More recent studies show largely similar results (Easterlin 2010, 2013, 2017; World Happiness Report 2016, 2021; Asadullah et al. 2018; Cheng et al. 2018; Clark et al. 2018; Diener et al. 2018; Frey and Stutzer 2018; Luo et al. 2018; Olivera 2019).[1]

---

[1] However, while "Havin' Money's Not Everything, Not Havin' It Is"; see Brzozowski and Spotton Visano (2020) on the importance of financial satisfaction.

When the above result was presented in a seminar, a colleague said, 'Cross-national relationship between income and happiness is affected by cultural differences. The relationship should be stronger within the same country.' In fact, the relationship between happiness and income level inter-temporally within the same country (at least for the advanced countries which have such data) is even less encouraging in terms of giving a positive relationship. For example, from the 1940s to 1994, the real income per capita of the US nearly trebled. However, the percentage of people who regard themselves as very happy fluctuated around 30%, without showing an upward trend; another measure of average happiness fluctuated around 72%. Since 1958, the real income level in Japan increased by more than 5 times. However, its average happiness measure fluctuated around 59%, also without an upward trend. (See Diener and Suh 1997; Frank 1997; Myers 1996, p. 445; Oswald 1997; Veenhoven 1993). Blanchflower and Oswald 2000 show that the levels of happiness in the United States have declined slightly over the period from the early 1970's to the late 1990's while (Hagerty and Veenhoven 1999) show a slight increase. 'Roughly unchanged' seems still to be the best bet.). Perhaps, dynamically, we need rising incomes just to sustain happiness at an unchanged level, the so-called 'hedonic treadmill'. However, there are also studies showing happiness to be *inversely* related to the pace of economic growth (Diener et al. 1993).

There could also be different degrees of cultural bias in reports of happiness levels internationally (Diener et al. 2009). For example, people in the US are more inclined to profess happiness, as being happy is socially regarded as something positive. French respondents may have the opposite bias, as Charles de Gaulle was quoted as saying *'Happy people are idiots'*, though this assertion has actually been refuted by evidence (Diener 1984). In Japan, the social custom of modesty may make people less ready to describe themselves as very happy. However, for intertemporal comparisons, it is likely that, if there have been any significant changes in such biases, they are likely towards more willingness to profess happiness. Thus, such cultural bias cannot be used to explain the failure of the happiness measures to increase over time with income. Moreover, researchers have used various methods (e.g. the social desirability scale of Crowne and Marlowe (1964) to isolate the effects of such biases without changing the conclusions significantly. For example, Konow and Earley (2002) report that the use of the C-M scale to control for the bias does not significantly affect their findings that people who help others are happier.

On the other hand, happiness studies show that a number of factors including marriage, personality, health, religious belief, employment, social capital correlate positively and strongly with happiness (e.g. Winkelmann and Winkelmann 1998; Bjornskov 2003; Diener et al. 2010; Amato and James 2018; Leng et al. 2020). For example, for personality, 'the most robust predictors of higher life satisfaction were higher extraversion, conscientiousness, emotional stability (lower neuroticism)' (Kobylińska et al. 2020, Abstract).

It is interesting that age correlates with happiness in an unexpected way. Most people may expect that happiness first increases with age as one gains more independence, incomes, and knowledge to enjoy life and then decreases with age as one gets old and less healthy. Happiness researchers first found no significant relationship between age and happiness. However, when they allow for the square of age in the regression, they find that average happiness first decreases with age until around thirty something years old and then increases monotonically with age until the highest range available in studies, seventy something. That the minimum point occurs at around thirty something could be explained by the pressure of paying off the first mortgage on the housing loan, inexperience in adjusting to one's partner and in bringing up the first child. Knowledge of this unexpected U-shaped happiness curve is very, very important, especially to the majority of readers of this book who may be around or will soon reach the minimum happiness point in their life cycles. Some of the less happy may think, 'I am already so unhappy at this young age; won't I have an even more miserable life when I am old? Perhaps I should end this miserable life!' The knowledge of the U-shaped happiness curve may thus prevent many suicides and provide a more optimistic outlook by knowing a brighter future ahead. This knowledge alone is certainly worth many, many times the total opportunity costs of buying and reading this book! Your happiness is also increased by knowing that your consumer surplus of buying this book is so huge; haha! (On the age-happiness relationship, see Chap. 9.)

The picture is not much different even if we use more objective indicators of the quality of life. Analyzing a panel data set of 95 quality-of-life indicators (covering education, health, transport, inequality, pollution, democracy, political stability) covering 1960–1990, Easterly (1999) reaches some remarkable results. While virtually all of these indicators show quality of life across nations to be positively associated with per capita income, when country effects are removed using either fixed effects or an estimator in first differences, the effects of economic growth on the quality of life are uneven and often nonexistent. It is found that *'quality of life is about equally likely to improve or worsen with rising income. ... In the sample of 69 indicators available for the irst Differences indicator, 62 percent of the indicators had time shifts improve the indicator more than growth did'* (Easterly 1999, p. 17–8). Even for the only 20 out of the 81 indicators with a significantly positive relationship with income under fixed effects, time improved 10 out of these 20 indicators more than income did.

The surprising results are not due to the worsening income distribution (there is some evidence that the share of the poor gets better with growth). Rather, the quality of life of any country depends less on its own economic growth or income level but more on the scientific, technological, and other breakthroughs at the world level. These depend more on public spending than private consumption (Radcliff 2013; Ott 2015; Ho et al. 2020; Cf. Dowding and Taylor 2020). Many studies (e.g. Estes 1988; Slottje 1991; see Offer 2000 for a review) show that measures of social progress strongly correlate with income level at low incomes (to around US$3,000 at 1981 prices) but the correlation disappears after that. Others (e.g. Veenhoven 1991; Diener and Suh 1999) show a similar relationship between happiness and income.

Higher income and consumption may increase the preference for even higher levels but they may in fact decrease the happiness level if the consumption level remains unchanged. In other words, higher consumption makes us adapted to the

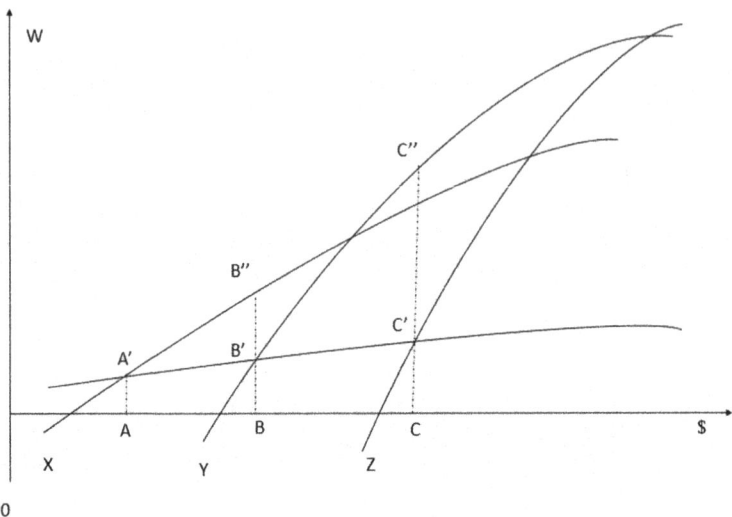

Fig. 7.1 The adaptation of happiness to customary consumption levels

higher level and raises our expectation and hence makes us needing even higher consumption to remain at the same welfare level. As illustrated in Fig. 7.1, when one's customary consumption level is indicated by the point A, the (total) welfare curve is X. When one's customary level increases to B, the curve moves to Y. Thus, the welfare level does not increase to BB" but only marginally to BB'. However, the marginal welfare of consumption (originally measured by the slope of the curve X at point A') may increase (to the slope of the curve Y at B'). This makes the individual feel that having more money to spend becomes more important. However, the long-run welfare curve is the curve that passes through A'B'C' which has a much lower slope, indicating that the marginal welfare of consumption is low. According to the estimate of Kapteyn et al. (1976), up to 80% of an expected initial welfare increase of additional income disappears with an actual increase in income. Fuentes and Rojas (2001) found that income does not have a strong influence on either well-being or on the probability of happiness. '*However, people tend to overstress the impact that additional income would have on their subjective well-being*'(p. 289).

If we take into account the costs of adjustment, the whole long-run welfare curve is also a function of one's accustomed level of consumption a higher level of which lowers the whole long-run welfare curve. To maximize happiness in the long run, one should start with not too high a consumption level so as to be able to gradually increase the level over time. In this perspective, children of the rich may really suffer a disadvantage. (This is supported by evidence on adolescents reported in Schneider, B., & Csikszentmihalyi 2000.) They start off being accustomed to very high levels of consumption which they may find difficult to surpass, hence suffering in happiness terms. Thus, wise rich people do not splash their children with money. But there are difficulties for the rich in limiting the consumption levels of their children, due to comparison with those of the parents and with peers. This may also partly explain why there is not much difference in happiness terms between the rich and the poor.

Failing to realize expectation is important in student examination performance. The despair after non-realization makes many students giving up, fail to pass, and drop out of school. An intervention to help students adjust to more realistic expectation reduce the failure/drop-out rates by 25–40% (Goux et al. 2017).

Reich (2000) argues for putting more time for one's family than in long working hours and is thus in agreement with the theme here. However, his proposal of providing US$60,000 for everyone turning 18 may not be a good idea as it is contrary to the principle of starting from a low consumption level as well as the merit of self-reliance.

There is a consideration that qualifies the above principle of starting from a low consumption level. For certain items of consumption, especially those important for health, too low a level does not only fail to improve one's future ability to happiness, it actually lowers that ability. This is especially so in one's childhood and adolescent periods where sufficient (material and spiritual) nutrients are important for the healthy growth of the body, the development of healthy personality, and the build up of knowledge (Glewwe et al. 2001). If one is handicapped by serious deficiencies earlier in life, one may never catch up later. However, this consideration is more important than the adaptation effect only at very low consumption levels. It may be thought that an informed and rational individual would know and take account of the long-run effects and hence the problem does not arise. However, the evidence suggests that most individuals are not perfectly rational and/or informed in this sense and that they are thus guided more by their short-run curves (Frijters 2000; Gilbert 2006; Shafir 2008; Linden 2011).

References

AMATO, P. R., & JAMES, S. L. (2018). Changes in spousal relationships over the marital life course,In: Alwin D., Felmlee D., Kreager D. (eds). *Social Networks and the Life Course*, Frontiers in Sociology and Social Research, vol 2. Springer, Cham,pp. 139–158. Available at:https://www.businessinsider.sg/happiest-point-in-marriage-2018-4/?r=US&IR=T

ASADULLAH, M. N., XIAO, S., & YEOH, E. (2018). Subjective well-being in China, 2005–2010: The role of relative income, gender, and location. *China Economic Review, 48*, 83–101.

BJORNSKOV, Christian. (2003). The happy few: Cross-country evidence on social capital and life satisfaction. *Kyklos, 56*(1), 3–16.

BLANCHFLOWER, David & OSWALD, Andrew (2000). Well-being over time in Britain and the USA, *Paper presented at Conference on Economics and the Pursuit of Happiness*, Nuffield College, Oxford University, February.

BRZOZOWSKI, M. & SPOTTON VISANO, B. (2020). "Havin' money's not everything, not havin' it is": The importance of financial satisfaction for Life satisfaction in financially stressed households. *Journal of Happiness Studies, 21*, 573–591. https://doi.org/10.1007/s10902-019-00091-0

CHENG, H., CHEN, C., LI, D., & YU, H. (2018). The mystery of Chinese people's happiness. *Journal of Happiness Studies, 19*(7), 2095–2114.

CLARK, A. E., FLÉCHE, S., LAYARD, R., POWDTHAVEE, N., & WARD, G. (2018). *The Origins of Happiness: The Science of Well-Being over the Life Course*. Princeton University Press.

CROWNE, D. P. and MARLOWE, D. A. (1964). *The Approval Motive: Studies in Evaluative Dependence*. Wiley.

CUMMINS, Robert A. (1998). The second approximation to an international standard for life satisfaction. *Social Indicators Research, 43*, 307–344.

DIENER, Ed. (1984). Subjective well-being. *Psychological Bulletin, 95*, 542–575.

DIENER, E., DIENER, M., DIENER, C. (2009). Factors Predicting the Subjective Well-Being of Nations. In DIENER, E. (eds), *Culture and Well-Being*, Social Indicators Research Series, 38. Springer, Dordrecht. https://doi.org/10.1007/978-90-481-2352-0_3.

DIENER, E., LUCAS, R. E., & OISHI, S. (2018). Advances and open questions in the science of subjective well-being. *Collabra: Psychology*, 4(1), 15. DOI: https://doi.org/10.1525/collabra.115.

DIENER, Ed & SUH, Eunkook (1997). Measuring quality of life: Economic, social and subjective indicators. *Social Indicators Research*, 40: 189–216.

DIENER, Ed & SUH, Eunkook (1999).National differences in subjective well-being.Chapter 22 in KAHNEMAN, D., DIENER, E. & SCHWARZ, N. *Well-being: The foundations of hedonic psychology* (pp. 434–450). New York, NY, US: Russell Sage Foundation.

DIENER, Ed, SANDVIK, Ed, SEIDLITS, Larry & DIENER, Marissa (1993). The relationship between income and subjective well-being: relative or absolute? *Social Indicators Research*, 28: 195–223.

DIENER, Ed., KAHNEMAN, Daniel. & HELLIWELL, John, F. (2010). *International Differences in Well-Being*. Oxford: Oxford University Press.

DOWDING, Keith and TAYLOR, Brad R. (2020). *Economic Perspectives on Government*. Foundations of Government and Public Administration.

EASTERLEY, William (1999), 'Life during growth', World Bank working paper. Available on web page: http://www.worldbank.org/html/prdmg/grthweb/growth_t.htmEASTERLIN, Richard A. (1974). Does economic growth improve the human lot? In P. A. David and M. W. Reder (Eds.), *Nations and Households in Economic Growth: Essays in Honour of Moses Abramovitz*. New York: Academic Press.

EASTERLIN, R. A., MCVEY, L. A., SWITEK, M., SAWANGFA, O., & ZWEIG, J. S. (2010). The happiness–income paradox revisited. *Proceedings of the National Academy of Sciences, 107*(52), 22463–22468.

EASTERLIN, Richard A. (2013). Happiness, growth, and public policy. *Economic Inquiry, 51*(1), 1–15.

EASTERLIN, Richard A. (2017). Paradox Lost?, *Review of Behavioral. Economics*, 4(4), 311–339. https://doi.org/10.1561/105.00000068

ESTES, Richard J. (1988). *Trends in World Social Development: The Social Progress of Nations, 1970–1987*. Praeger.

FRANK, R. H. (1997). Conspicuous consumption: Money well spent? *Journal of Economic, 107*, 1832–1847.

FREY, Bruno S. (2018). Psychological influences on happiness. In FREY, Bruno S., and Alois STUTZER. *Economics of Happiness*. Springer, Cham., pp. 25–27.

FRIJTERS, Paul. (2000). Do individuals try to maximize general satisfaction? *Journal of Economic Psychology, 21*(3), 281–304.

FUENTES, Nicole & ROJAS, Mariano. (2001). Economic theory and subjective well-being: Mexico. *SIR, 53*(3), 289–314.

GILBERT, D. (2006). *Stumbling on Happiness*. Knopf.

GLEWWE, Paul, JACOBY, Hanan G. & KING Elizabeth. (2001). 'Early childhood nutrition and academic achievement: a longitudinal analysis', *Journal of Public Economics*, 81(3):345-368.

GOUX, D. et al. (2017). Adjusting your dream? *Economic Journal*, 1025–46.

HAGERTY, Michael R. & VEENHOVEN, Ruut (1999), 'Wealth and happiness revisited: growing wealth of nations does go with greater happiness', Typescript.

References

HO, Lok Sang, et al. (2020). Happiness and government: The role of public spending and public governance, manuscript.

INGLEHART, Ronald, BASNEZ, Miguel & MORENO, Alejandro. (1998). *Human Values and Beliefs: A Cross-Cultural Sourcebook: Political, Religious, Sexual, and Economic Norms in 43 Societies; Findings from the 1990–1993 World Value Survey*. University of Michigan Press.

KAPTEYN, A., VAN PRAAG, B.M.S. & VAN HERWAARDEN, F.G. (1976). 'Individual welfare functions and social reference spaces', *E. Letters, 1*, 173–178.

KOBYLIŃSKA, D., ZAJENKOWSKI, M., LEWCZUK, K. et al. (2020). The mediational role of emotion regulation in the relationship between personality and subjective well-being. *Current Psychology*. https://doi.org/10.1007/s12144-020-00861-7

KONOW, James and EARLEY, Joseph (2002). *The hedonistic paradox: is homo economics happier?* unpublished manuscript.

LENG, X., HAN, J., ZHENG, Y. et al. (2020). The Role of a "Happy Personality" in the Relationship of Subjective Social Status and Domain-Specific Satisfaction in China. *Applied Research Quality Life*. https://doi.org/10.1007/s11482-020-09839-w

LINDEN, David J. (2011). *The Compass of Pleasure*. Viking.

LUO, Yangmei, WANG, Tong, and HUANG, Xiting (2018) . Which types of income matter most for well-being in China: Absolute, relative or income aspirations? *International Journal of Psychology, 53*(3): 218–222.

MYERS, David. (1996). *Social Psychology*. Macmillan.

OFFER, Avner (2000). Economic welfare measurements and human well-being. University of Oxford Discussion Papers in Economic and Social History, No. 34.

OLIVERA, S.V. (2019). Review of *Happiness, Wellbeing and Society. What Matters for Singaporeans* by TAMBYAH, Siok Kuan & TAN, Soo Jiuan,*Applied Research Quality Life*, doi:https://doi.org/10.1007/s11482-019-09737-w

OSWALD, Andrew J. (1997). Happiness and economic performance. *The Economic Journal, 107*, 1815–1831.

OTT, Jan C. (2015). Impact of size and quality of governments on happiness: Financial insecurity as a key-problem in market-democracies. *Journal of Happiness Studies, 16*, 1639–1647.

RADCLIFF, Benjamin (2013) *The Political Economy of Human Happiness*, Cambridge University Press.

REICH, Robert (2000/1), *The Future of Success*. Vintage.

SCHNEIDER, B. & CSIKSZENTMIHALYI, M. (2000). *Becoming adult: How teenagers prepare for the world of work*. New York: Basic Books.

SHAFIR, E. (2008). A Behavioral perspective on consumer protection. *Competition and Consumer Law Journal, 15*(3), 302–317.

SLOTTJE, Daniel (1991). *Measuring the Quality of Life across Countries: A Multidimensional Analysis*. Boulder, Col.: Westview.

VEENHOVEN, Ruut. (1991). Is happiness relative? *Social Indicators Research, 24*, 1–34.

VEENHOVEN, Ruut (1993). *Happiness in Nations: Subjective Appreciation of Life in 56 Nations 1946–1992*. Rotterdam: RISBO.

VEENHOVEN, Ruut & TIMMERMANS, D. (1998). *Welvaart en geluk*, ESB (Dutch).

WINKELMANN, Liliana & WINKELMANN, Rainer. (1998). Why are the unemployed so unhappy? *Economica, 65*, 1–15.

World Happiness Report (2016, 2018, 2019, 2020). Retrieved from: https://worldhappiness.report/ed/2020/.

Open Access This chapter is licensed under the terms of the Creative Commons Attribution 4.0 International License (http://creativecommons.org/licenses/by/4.0/), which permits use, sharing, adaptation, distribution and reproduction in any medium or format, as long as you give appropriate credit to the original author(s) and the source, provide a link to the Creative Commons license and indicate if changes were made.

The images or other third party material in this chapter are included in the chapter's Creative Commons license, unless indicated otherwise in a credit line to the material. If material is not included in the chapter's Creative Commons license and your intended use is not permitted by statutory regulation or exceeds the permitted use, you will need to obtain permission directly from the copyright holder.

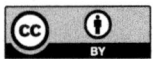

Chapter 8
Environmentally Responsible Happy Nation Index: A Proposed National Success Indicator

Abstract The average happy life years HLY (of a country) is the product of the average happiness (or life satisfaction) index and the life expectancy index. Adjusting HLY to get rid of the misleading parts with negative happiness to obtain the adjusted or net HLY; deducting again the per-capita environmental costs imposed on others, we obtain the 'environmentally responsible happy nation index' as an internationally acceptable national success indicator that accounts positively for long and happy lives but negatively at the external costs of environmental disruption imposed on others and in the future. Hopefully, this 'environmentally responsible happy nation index' will lead to some re-orientation of both the market and national governments towards something more fundamentally valuable.

8.1 Introduction

For many decades, some measures of national income (GDP, GNP and its per capita values) have been used as a comprehensive achievement or success indicator of a nation, at least in the economic sphere. The inadequacy of such income measures prompts the development of improvements or alternative measures, including the proposals in the 1970's for taking account of leisure time and pollution, a 'genuine progress indicator' (Halstead 1998; Hamilton 1998), a 'measure of domestic progress' (Jackson 2004), and the launching by the United Nations of the Human Development Report in 1990 (which provides the Human Development Index, the Gender-related Development Index, the Gender Empowerment Measure, and the Human Poverty Index). The Human Development Index combines indices of life expectancy, education, and PPP-adjusted GDP per capita. While such indices are certainly relevant, they are still inadequate. Thus, it is 'perfectly possible … to be well-educated, free of illness and rich, but miserable and lonely' (Marks et al. 2006, p. 6).

As happiness is the only intrinsic value, ultimately speaking (Chap. 5), and as economic growth no longer increase happiness significantly after a rather low level of survival and comfort (Chap. 7), it is natural that we should look for a largely happiness-based index. Thus, the focus on happiness and its relationships with economic and other variables by economists since the commencement of this century (e.g. Frey and Stutzer 2002a; Layard 2005; van Praag & Ferrer-i-Carbonell 2004; Di Tella and MacCulloch 2006) is to be welcome. Sociologists and other researchers have also devised various measures of quality of life (QOL) indicators (see Hagerty et al. 2001 for a review and a set of criteria for evaluating the indexes, and Ridzi et al. 2020 for some recent discussion). However, as emphasized by Hajiran (2006, pp. 33–4), 'Improving QOL is just "a means" and not "an end" in itself. The ultimate goal of improving QOL is to maintain and enhance the scope, depth and intensity of human well-being or "happiness"'. Thus, good QOL indicators should reflect this ultimate goal. More subjective indices have also been proposed, from Andrews and Withey (1976) and Campbell et al. (1976) to Diener (2000), Cummins et al. (2003), and Kahneman et al. (2004), Tanaka and Tokimatsu (2020).

For an individual, happiness or welfare[1] is probably the most important ultimate objective. However, at the national and global level and for the welfare of the future, we have to consider two related factors, the possible costs imposed on others and the sustainability of the situation. The most important variable here is the environmental disruption imposed on our life support systems.

We do not really want just a single index. For different purposes, different indices may be relevant (Cf. Ruggeri et al. 2020). For example, even just for purely economic production, even after we know the GDP figure, we may still want to know the figure for say total output of cars. On the other hand, some indices could certainly be improved. For example, the gross material production index used by the former centrally planned economies that involves double counting over different stages of production (e.g. wheat, flour, and bread all counted at their full values, not just values added) but that excludes services can be seen to be inferior to the modern concept of national income or product. The former index had thus been discarded.

It is the purpose of this chapter to propose some improvements over certain measures and to advance a measure of national success indicator that takes into account the ultimate objective of life and the external costs imposed on others and on the future. In particular, this chapter argues that.

- Existing method of calculating the measure of happy life years should be revised to give a more accurate figure (Sect. 8.3).
- A revised index called the environmentally responsible happy nation index (ERHNI) is proposed as an internationally more acceptable national success indicator (Sect. 8.4) and calculated for the various countries with the relevant data (Sect. 8.5).
- ERHNI = revised HLY - per capita external costs.

---

[1] These two terms are used interchangeably here. In everyday usage, happiness probably refers to current situation while welfare refers to the long term. For any given time period, the two are the same. If I am very happy over a certain period, my welfare over that period must be high. On the other hand, 'utility' which represents 'preference' may differ from happiness due to ignorance (including imperfect foresight), a concern for the welfare of others, and imperfect rationality; see Chap. 2.

8.2 Revising the Measurement of Happy Life Years

Since happiness (or other similar measures like life satisfaction) is measured for a given period (like a week or a year) but an individual may live a short or a long live, the happiness index itself does not give the total amount of happiness enjoyed over the whole lifespan. The concept of happy life years (Veenhoven) is conceived to overcome this problem. Conceptually, HLY is just the product of the average happiness index over the lifespan and the length of the lifespan (of life expectancy). For any given average happiness level (if positive), everyone would like to live a longer than a shorter life. Thus, HLY is an important extension of the measurement of happiness. However, an important revision in the actual measurement of HLY is needed.

As measured by Veenhoven (2005), happy-life-years = happiness (index in the range of 0–1) times life-expectancy at birth (in years). The happiness index is converted from the normal index in the range 0–100 or 0–10 into 0–1, e.g. an index of 50 (out of 100) is converted into 0.5. This measure has the following problem. It is well known that, for a scale of 0–10, the figure of 5 typically corresponds to the level of neutrality in net happiness. Since the level of overall net happiness can be either positive or negative (an individual can be happy or unhappy), and since the figure of 50% is typically used as the bare passing grade in schools, most people also habitually use the figure of 5 out of 10 or 50 out of 100 to represent the level of zero net happiness as is also the case for the curve in Fig. 1.1. (Some surveys explicitly locate the neutrality point at 5.) The average happiness indices of most nations in the world fall within the range of 4 to 8 (out of 10).

Consider the following two situations:

- A. An average happiness index of 4 (out of 10) with a lifespan of 100, giving a HLY index of 40 (with the happiness index normalized to the range 0–1 as in Veenhoven's measure);
- B. An average happiness index of 6.5 (out of 10) with a lifespan of 60, giving a HLY index of 39.

Which situation or life experience would you rather have? Since an index of 5 means neutrality (neither happy nor unhappy), the index of 4 really mean unhappiness, with negative net happiness, or unhappiness more than happiness. For such a life, it is better to have a shorter than a longer life, as a longer life really mean longer suffering. Thus, most people will definitely choose B over A. However, existing measure of HLY rank A higher than B. This is very misleading.

This difficulty can be easily overcome. We should count only the value over neutrality as being valuable. In the above example, the adjusted HLY for the two situations are calculated as:

A. $(4-5)$ times 0.1 (conversion to the scale of 0–1) times $100 = -10$ (minus ten).
B. $(6.5-5)$ times 0.1 times $60 = 9$.

The superiority of B over A can then be reflected by the positive index of 9 for B over the negative figure of minus 10 for A.

Without the above adjustment, the problem still remains even if no happiness index below the neutrality level of 5 is involved. Consider:

- C. An average happiness index of 5.1 with a lifespan of 100, giving an unadjusted HLY index of 51.
- D. An average happiness index of 8 with a lifespan of 60, giving an unadjusted HLY index of 48.

Again, most people would rather have a very happy life of 60 years rather than a barely worth living life of 100 years. The adjusted HLY gives:

- C: $(5.1 - 5)$ times 0.1 times $100 = 1$.
- D: $(8 - 5)$ times 0.1 times $60 = 18$.

This shows a clear superiority of D over C as consistent with the preferences of most people, as well as with rationality.

If the above adjustment is done, is the adjusted HLY an appropriate national success indicator?

8.3 Towards an International Acceptable National Success Indicator

For an individual, ignoring the effects on others, the adjusted HLY seems an appropriate indicator. However, for a whole nation, if say America is able to achieve a very high adjusted HLY, but only by imposing very high environmental costs, making people in other countries and in the future suffer enormously, this is not a good outcome. (On the importance of the natural environment for happiness, see Chaps. 5 and 6, World Happiness Report 2020.) Thus, to provide an appropriate national success indicator, it seems natural to allow for the adjusted HLY positively, and the (per-capita) net external costs imposed on others negatively. In principle, the net external costs may account for the balance of various external costs and benefits. Due to the overwhelming importance of environmental protection, we may concentrate on the costs of environmental disruption. We then have the environmentally responsible happy nation index (ERHNI) as our proposed national success indicator,

ERHNI = Adjusted HLY—per capita external costs

where ERHNI = Environmentally Responsible Happy Nation Index.[2]

---

[2] A possible issue is whether the equality in happiness should be taken into account. In my view, inequality in income is undesirable both because of the diminishing marginal utility of income and because of the indirect undesirable effects of inequality in reducing happiness through for example reducing social cohesion. Since happiness is already the ultimate objective, we can neither have diminishing marginal happiness of happiness nor further indirect effects, except in an intertemporal framework where the happiness in the future has not yet been accounted for. (Correctly accounting for this intertemporal effect, an objective function that is not linear in individual happiness can be shown to violate some compelling axiom, i.e. treating a perceptible increment of happiness as less

8.3 Towards an International Acceptable National Success Indicator

The index for per capita external costs measures the aggregate costs imposed on the global community by the nation concerned in per capita terms. Note that the 'per capita' here is in the sense of per person within the home nation. Thus, if a nation of 1 billion persons imposes a total environmental costs on the rest of the world (including the future) equivalent to 6 billion Adjusted HLY, its per capita external cost is not 0.1 (6 billion/60 billion) but rather 6 (6 billion/1 billion). Thus, ERHNI measures the amount of happy life years a nation achieves for an average person less the per capita costs imposed externally on the global community. A nation that achieves a high HLY and a low PCEC (and hence a high ERHNI) not only entails high happy life years for its own residents but also imposes low (per capita) costs externally (on others). Since the main form of external costs is probably environmental disruption, the index is called 'environmentally responsible happy nation index' (ERHNI). If ERHNI is accepted as a measure of national success, governments and people in different nations around the world will not only each strive to achieve a high level of HLY but will also strive to lower the costs imposed on others. This will enhance the ability of each nation to achieve a high HLY index and the ability of the world to sustain a high HLY more permanently.

If we sum the two terms (on the right hand side of the above equation) to get ERHNI, the two terms have to be in comparable units. Since the relevant external costs are on the whole world including the effects in the future, we cannot expect to have a very accurate estimate. However, starting with some imperfect estimates (or even just guestimates) may have the advantage of leading to more accurate estimates. It is better to be roughly right on important things than to be perfectly accurate on things that are irrelevant. Since environmental disruption is clearly a very important issue that may even threaten our survival, it is imperative that we have some national success indicator that gives sufficient recognition of the negative environmental costs. The concept of green GDP takes some account of this. However, recent happiness studies (see summaries in e.g. Frey and Stutzer 2002a; Layard 2005; Kahneman and Krueger 2006; Ahuvia 2008; Asadullah et al. 2018; Cheng et al. 2018; Luo et al. 2018; Sherman et al. 2020) show that, at the social level (where individual relative competition cancels out) incomes above a relatively low level does not increase happiness (at least not to any significant extent). Thus, income is inferior to happiness as the ultimate national success indicator. Secondly, depending on the particular method of adjustment (from the traditional GDP), the measure of green GDP may mainly emphasize the environmental effects on the country concerned, while the concept of ERHNI emphasize the costs imposed on others and the future. Also, though we propose to start with environmental costs, the concept of external costs in ERHNI need not be confined to environmental costs. Once we shift from income to happiness, the environmental costs internal to the country concerned is already largely reflected in the measure of HLY of that country, though some effects on the

---

important than a less than a perceptible one; see Ng 1975, 1984.) Moreover, the argument for the utilitarian social welfare function (Ng 2000, Chap. 5; also Chap. 5) supports not taking into account inequality in the ultimate objective. Also, Ott (2005) shows that higher average happiness tends to go with higher equality in happiness.

future may still not be fully captured. Thus, for the measure of ERHNI, we focus on the environmental costs external to that nation and imposed on the world.

What should be included under external costs could be further discussed. However, we may start with the global environmental costs imposed by a nation. Before a more comprehensive measure of PCEC or its main component per capita global environmental costs has been calculated, Ng (2008) uses the figures for CO_2 emissions calculated by the United Nations' Department of Economic and Social Affairs as the proxy. This is based on the reasoning that the most important global environmental cost is probably that of global warming which is threatening the sustainability of the whole life support system of the whole world. CO_2 is the principal greenhouse gas. Thus, using CO_2 emissions may be a better proxy for external costs than the full ecological footprint which includes both external and non-external items. In any case, our calculation is mainly illustrative. When a more appropriate figure for the external cost index is available, it could be used instead.

8.4 Estimating the Environmentally Responsible Happy Nation Index

The Environmentally Responsible Happy Nation Index (ERHNI) may be estimated for the various nations in the world if sufficient data are available. If we wait until we have perfect data, we will wait forever. Partly for the purpose of illustration and partly to kick start the endeavour, I calculated the ERHNI indices for 142 countries with available data (in 2006) based on very rough estimates of the relevant variables in Ng (2008), which should be consulted on the detailed method of estimation. Here only some of the results are reported.

The results show that nations with low ERHNI indices are mainly African and former communist countries (with their poverty and difficulties of transition, respectively),[3] due more to their low life satisfaction figures than their high external costs. In Asia, only Pakistan has a negative figure and no nation in Western Europe and (North and Latin) Americas has a negative index. This is partly because our estimate of PCEC is conservative or has a significantly downward bias. However, although our conservative estimate of external costs does not turn the ERHNI of these nations into a negative figure, it nevertheless gives a different picture than just the figures for HLY. For example, in North America, Canada and the USA have very similar values in terms of life satisfaction, but Canada has an ERHNI value (11.3) significantly higher that of the USA (8.064) due to a lower per capita total CO_2 emission (and hence our estimate of PCEC) of Canada than USA. Nations in Western Europe which mostly have emission figures even lower than Canada, register high ERHNI figures, taking six out of the top ten nations reported in Table 8.1, with Switzerland and Denmark heading the list. Leading nations in the Asia–Pacific area are New

---

[3] On the negative effects of transition on happiness, especially for Poland and Russia, see Brzezinski (2019).

8.4 Estimating the Environmentally Responsible Happy Nation Index

Table 8.1 Top scores in ERHNI, 2008 estimates

	Country	ERHNI
	WORLD	
	Weighted Average	**4.705**
1	Switzerland	22.789
2	Denmark	19.339
3	Costa Rica	18.745
4	Sweden	18.534
5	Austria	17.536
6	Panama	15.430
7	Colombia	15.261
8	Netherlands	14.963
9	Ireland	14.716
10	Venezuela	14.533
	ASIA–PACIFIC	
	Average	**5.158**
1	New Zealand	14.304
2	Malaysia	14.167
3	Indonesia	9.967
4	Philippines	9.346
5	Mongolia	9.240

Zealand, Malaysia, Indonesia, Philippines, and Mongolia, as listed in the lower part of Table 8.1. A table reporting the results for all the 142 countries is in Ng (2008). (This has been extended and updated by Chen et al. (2016) the result of which is reported in Table 8.2.)

Following Ng (2008), Chen et al. (2016) make some important refinements to the proposed ERHNI and use wider (than just CO_2) scope for external costs and also using more updated (2015) data and have a new estimate for an expanded set of 151 countries. Only the top 15 scorers are reported in Table 8.2.

8.5 Concluding Remarks

It is true that the existing happiness or life satisfaction measures are not perfectly accurate and the external costs measures are also very rudimentary and incomplete. However, we did not wait for the measure of GNP to be improved by the green adjustments, the PPP adjustments, etc. before using it. We also did not wait for the measures of happiness and life satisfaction to be perfected before using them. Recent happiness studies show that income is a poor correlate with happiness (Chap. 7), especially at the social level. Our ultimate objective is really happiness rather than

Table 8.2 Top 15 Scorers in Chen et al. (2016) ERHNI Rankings

Country	Well-being (0–10)	Life expectancy	Adjusted or net HLY	Ext Cost Ratio	PCEC	ERHNI
Denmark	7.8	80.05121951	22.17831272	0.001254709971	0.3094890627	21.86882366
Canada	7.7	81.23804878	21.5308959	0.002646939606	0.6528989781	20.87799692
Switzerland	7.5	82.69756098	20.87716992	0.0005603911507	0.1382271091	20.73894281
Norway	7.6	81.45121951	21.44030312	0.002965036758	0.731361405	20.70894172
Sweden	7.5	81.70487805	20.39369332	0.001016711812	0.2507840003	20.14290932
Netherlands	7.5	81.10487805	20.29143346	0.001086636558	0.2680317663	20.02340169
Israel	7.4	81.70487805	19.27349526	0.00039630003742	0.09775217716	19.17574309
Finland	7.4	80.62682927	19.29613046	0.001485188531	0.3663393272	18.92979114
Austria	7.3	80.93658537	18.98801396	0.0008923687237	0.2201133061	18.76790065
Australia	7.4	82.04634146	19.7372004	0.004754715091	1.172806745	18.56439365
Costa Rica	7.3	79.70502439	18.10143991	0.0004248598118	0.1047967004	17.99664321
Venezuela	7.5	74.4875122	18.46139003	0.001666053473	0.4109518053	18.05043822
Panama	7.3	77.36809756	17.96075233	0.0007676484744	0.1893495806	17.77140274
Ireland	7.3	80.89512195	18.26118106	0.002691532484	0.663898339	17.59728272
United States of America	7.2	78.74146341	17.03663054	0.001520823025	0.3751289967	16.66150155

incomes. Thus, having a measure of national success in terms of some appropriate measure of happiness is very important. Moreover, just shifting to happiness alone is not sufficient. If each of the 200 or so nations in the world strives to increase the happiness level of its own people without sufficient check on the external costs imposed on the rest of the world, we may still have the tragedy of the commons.

A desirable national success indicator should take into account not only the (average) happy live years achieved for its own people, but must also take into (negative) account the external costs (only global environmental disruption is taken into account in this chapter, but the concept could be extended) imposed on others (including the future). The Environmentally Responsible Happy Nation Index (ERHNI) is proposed to serve this purpose. The calculation of this for the various nations reported in the last section is based on very rough and incomplete estimates. Nevertheless, it is hoped that, with further improvements, it will lead to some re-orientation of both the market and national governments towards something more fundamentally valuable and less damaging to our life support system.

References

AHUVIA, Aaron. (2008). If money doesn't make us happy, why do we act as if it does? *Journal of Economic Psychology, 29*, 491–507.
ANDREWS, Frank M. & WITHEY, Stephen B. (1976). *Social Indicators of Well-Being: American's Perceptions of Life Quality*. Plenum Press.
ASADULLAH, M. N., XIAO, S., & YEOH, E. (2018). Subjective well-being in China, 2005–2010: The role of relative income, gender, and location. *China Economic Review, 48*, 83–101.
BRZEZINSKI, M. (2019). Diagnosing Unhappiness Dynamics: Evidence from Poland and Russia. *Journal of Happiness Studies, 20*, 2291–2327. https://doi.org/10.1007/s10902-018-0044-6
CAMPBELL, Angus, CONVERSE, Philip. E. & RODGERS, Willard L. (1976). *The Quality of American Life: Perceptions, Evaluations, and Satisfactions*. Russell Sage Foundation.
CHEN, Enjiao, NG, Yew-Kwang, TAN, Yu Fen, TOH, Jesselyn Shi Ying. (2016). Environmentally responsible happy nation index: Refinements and 2015 rankings. *Social Indicators Research*. https://doi.org/10.1007/s11205-016-1422-2
CHENG, H., CHEN, C., LI, D., & YU, H. (2018). The mystery of Chinese people's happiness. *Journal of Happiness Studies, 19*(7), 2095–2114.
CUMMINS, Robert A., ECKERSLEY, Richard, PALLANT, Julie, VAN VUGT, Jackie & MISAJON, Rose Anne. (2003). Developing a national index of subjective wellbeing: The Australian Unity Wellbeing Index. *Social Indicators Research, 64*, 159–190.
DIENER, Ed (2000). Subjective well-being: the science of happiness and a proposal for a national index. *American Psychologist*, 55: 34–43.
DI TELLA, Rafael & MACCULLOCH, Robert (2006). Some uses of happiness data in economics. *Journal of Economic Perspectives, 20*(1), 25–46.
FREY, Bruno S. & STUTZER, Alois. (2002). *Happiness and Economics: How the Economy and Institutions Affect Well-Being*. Princeton University Press.
HAGERTY, Michael R., CUMMINS, Robert A., FERRISS, Abbott L., LAND, Kenneth, MICHALOS, Alex C., PETERSON, Mark, SHARPE, Andrew, SIRGY, Joseph & VOGEL, Joachim. (2001). Quality of Life Indexes for National Policy: Review and Agenda for Research. *Social Indicators Research, 55*(1), 1–96.
HAJIRAN, Homayoun. (2006). Toward a quality of life theory: Net domestic product of happiness. *Social Indicators Research, 75*(1), 31–43.

HALSTEAD, T. (1998). The science and politics of new measures of progress: A United States perspective. In R. Eckersley (Ed.), *Measuring Progress: Is Life Getting Better?* (pp. 53–68). CSIRO Publishing.

HAMILTON, C. (1998). Measuring changes in economic welfare: The genuine progress indicator for Australia. In R. Eckersley (Ed.), *Measuring Progress: Is Life Getting Better?* (pp. 69–92). CSIRO Publishing.

JACKSON, Tim. (2004). *Chasing Progress: Beyond Measuring Economic Growth.* New Economic Foundation.

KAHNEMAN, Daniel & KRUEGER, Alan B. (2006). Developments in the measurement of subjective well-being. *Journal of Economic Perspectives, 20*(1), 3–24.

KAHNEMAN, Daniel, KRUEGER, Alan B., SCHKADE, David, SCHWARTZ, Norbert & STONE, Arthur. (2004). Toward national well-being accounts. *American Economic Review, 94*(2), 429–434.

LAYARD, Richard. (2005). *Happiness: Lessons from a New Science.* Penguin.

LUO, Yangmei, WANG, Tong, and HUANG, Xiting. (2018). Which types of income matter most for well-being in China: Absolute, relative or income aspirations? *International Journal of Psychology, 53*(3), 218–222.

MARKS, Nic, et al. (2006), *The Happy Planet Index.* London: New Economics Foundation. Available at http://www.happyplanetindex.org

NG, Yew-Kwang. (1975). Bentham or Bergson? Finite sensibility, utility functions, and social welfare functions. *Review of Economic Studies, 42,* 545–570.

NG, Yew-Kwang. (1984). Expected subjective utility: Is the Neumann-Morgenstern utility the same as the neoclassical's? *Social Choice and Welfare, 1*(3), 177–186.

NG, Yew-Kwang. (2000). *Efficiency, Equality, and Public Policy: With a Case for Higher Public Spending.* Macmillan.

NG, Yew-Kwang. (2008). Environmentally responsible happy nation index. *Social Indicators Research, 85,* 425–446.

OTT, Jan. (2005). Level and inequality of happiness in nations: Does greater happiness of a greater number imply greater inequality in happiness? *Journal of Happiness Studies, 6*(4), 397–420.

RIDZI, Frank, STEVENS, Chantal & DAVERN, Melanie (2020). *Community Quality-of-Life Indicators,* Springer.

RUGGERI, K., GARCIA-GARZON, E., MAGUIRE, Á. et al. (2020). Well-being is more than happiness and life satisfaction: A multidimensional analysis of 21 countries. *Health and Quality of Life Outcomes, 18,* 192. https://doi.org/10.1186/s12955-020-01423-y

SHERMAN, A., SHAVIT, T. & BAROKAS, G. (2020). A dynamic model on happiness and exogenous wealth shock: The case of lottery winners. *Journal of Happiness Studies, 21*(1), 117–137. https://doi.org/10.1007/s10902-019-00079-w

TANAKA, S. and TOKIMATSU, K. (2020). Social capital, subjective well-being, and happiness: Evidence from a survey in various European and Asian countries to address the Stiglitz report. *Modern Economy, 11,* 322–348. https://doi.org/10.4236/me.2020.112026

VAN PRAAG, Bernard & FERRER-I-CARBONELL, Ada (2004). *Happiness Quantified: A Satisfaction Calculus Approach.* Oxford University Press.

VEENHOVEN, Ruut. (1996). Happy life-expectancy: A comprehensive measure of quality-of-life in Nations. *Social Indicators Research, 39,* 1–58.

Open Access This chapter is licensed under the terms of the Creative Commons Attribution 4.0 International License (http://creativecommons.org/licenses/by/4.0/), which permits use, sharing, adaptation, distribution and reproduction in any medium or format, as long as you give appropriate credit to the original author(s) and the source, provide a link to the Creative Commons license and indicate if changes were made.

The images or other third party material in this chapter are included in the chapter's Creative Commons license, unless indicated otherwise in a credit line to the material. If material is not included in the chapter's Creative Commons license and your intended use is not permitted by statutory regulation or exceeds the permitted use, you will need to obtain permission directly from the copyright holder.

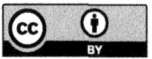

Chapter 9
Age and Happiness

Abstract Contrary to the common belief that the age-happiness relationship is mountain shape (the middle aged being happier than children and the aged), it is really largely U shape, with the middle aged (at around mid 30's or 40's) least happy. The increase from around 60 to 70's is particularly clear. However, happiness becomes lower over the last few years of illness before passing away. The decline in happiness from around 12 years old and the trough in happiness level around middle ages may partly be explained by the delay in sleep–wake cycles of teenagers, causing conflict with their mostly middle-aged parents. Recognizing the evolutionary ultimate explanation for this delay advanced here, the society should delay start hours for high schools to fit in with the delayed biological clock of teenagers.

9.1 The U-shape Relation of Age and Happiness

What is the relationship of age and happiness? Many if not most people (myself included before I looked at the evidence) believe that happiness should first mostly with age up to around the middle age, and then decline with age; the relationship is that of an inverted U shape, or mountain shape. This is thought to be so because children do not have independence, have the pressure of passing exam, and are not capable of enjoying life much; in contrast, the elderly have health problems and likely have lower incomes as well.

Actually, many studies in different countries discover that the situation is actually the opposite. Young children are fairly happy, and happiness starts to decline from around 11–12 years old (González-Carrasco et al. 2017). Happiness reaches a low at around mid-thirties to fifty something; then it increases (Gerdham and Johannesson 2001; Mroczek and Spiro 2005; Deaton 2008; Blanchflower and Oswald 2008; 2017; Cheng et al. 2017; Graham and Pozuelo 2017; Beja 2018; Laaksonen 2018; Butkovic et al. 2020), but decreases over the last few years (Fukuda 2013; Burns et al. 2014), typically with serious illness that ends their lives. A study on China shows the lowest point at around 34 years old (Graham et al. 2017).

Knowing this somewhat counter-intuitive evidence is very important. When you are very unhappy at say around early thirties, you may think that, I am young and healthy, but I am already so unhappy; won't it be horrible when I become old and unhealthy? Perhaps I should end this miserable life! Now, having known that the age-happiness relationship is largely U shape instead of mountain shape, when you are at your low, you will know that this is only the low point in life, and the future will be much better. Just this knowledge will reduce your unhappiness then and help you endure over that, instead of ending your life unwisely. This knowledge may thus save your life and increase your happiness. This is certainly worth many thousands of times the costs of reading this book.

Is the U shape relationship of age and happiness non-controversial? There were some controversies. Earlier, happiness researchers believed that there is no regular relationship between age and happiness; the happiness levels of individuals in different age groups are largely the same; on average, a person over different ages also has largely similar happiness levels. Differences and fluctuations are not mainly age-related, with no definite tendencies or patterns. They believed in this probably because there are many factors affecting happiness, with large interpersonal differences. In the absence of a large amount of data, it is very difficult to see any tendency or pattern. In later studies, with much more data, more reliable conclusions could be reached. For example, Blanchflower and Oswald (2017), using seven data sets from 51 countries covering 1.3 million randomly selected individuals from 20 to 90 years old, reaching the reliable conclusion that the age-happiness relationship is largely U shape.

I have read many papers on this issue and may safely conclude that, if we exclude the last few years of illness before death, in most cases, we do have the largely U shape age-happiness relationship. There are also some double U or W shape relationships. For example, a recent U.K. primary data set shows a low at around age 20, recovering to about 34 years old, and then declining to another low around 46; after 50, happiness recovers strongly until 70's. The U.S. data are similar, especially the jump in happiness from 60 to the 70's is very clear. Confucius said, 'I started to devote myself to study at the age of 15; became independent at 30; had no more illusions at 40; knew the mandate of Heaven at 50; could accept different opinions calmly at 60; could do whatever I want without overstepping any bounds at 70' (my translation). It was likely that his happiness also increased in the later few decades of his life.

An evidence strongly supporting that (net) happiness is U shape in age is that negative feelings and behavior like pressures, psychological problems, depressions, suicide rates, etc. are strongly mountain shape in age. These data are more objective and reliable. As these factors are strongly negatively related to happiness, this mountain shape supports the U shape age-happiness relationship. The Graham et al. (2017) study on China that reaches the lowest happiness level at around 34 years old, also shows a peak in these negative factors at around 33 years old.

Yet another interesting supporting evidence is from apes (including chimpanzees and orangutangs). Those feeding these apes can tell whether they are happy or unhappy from their appearance and behavior. Their happiness indices so judged are also U shape, with a low in middle age (Weiss et al. 2012).

9.1 The U-shape Relation of Age and Happiness

Why does our happiness initially fall with age to a trough at middle age and recover after that?

The decline in happiness from about age 12 is probably associated with puberty. Children at such ages start to have their own views which may be different from the parents. For example, some want to dye their hair into different colors and may have strong disputes with parents. They start to be interested in the opposite sex, but have little experience in relationship. Who they are interested in may not reciprocate. The pressure of study is also increasing.

The unhappiness at around 30's or 40's may be associated with financial pressures such as paying back housing loans, higher family responsibilities and expenses. It may also be the time pressure, with the need to take care of both the parents and children, at a time when working is important. Alternatively, it may also be due to being newly wed, still lacking experience in handling the relationship well; or first having a child, with no experience in caring for it. On the other hand, the higher happiness of the old may be due to the higher wisdom, and like Confucius, being able to do as one wishes without overstepping bounds.[1] However, for my case, though I have long known the mandate of Heaven (well, well over 50), I still have illusions. If I do as I want, I will certainly be put into prison. Nevertheless, my own happiness levels also conform to the general pattern, being U shape with age. My least happy period was also in my early thirties. Since then, my happiness increased every decade, with the peak at the current decade in my 70's.

I have an observation that may partly explain the decrease in and the low happiness level of teenagers and those in their middle ages simultaneously, as well as a simple way to increase their happiness. This is related to the delay in the sleep/wake cycle of teenagers, as discussed below.

9.2 The Delay in Sleep/wake Cycles of Teenagers: Ultimate Reason and Implications

We are all familiar with the sleep/wake cycle. This basic circadian rhythms of day-night wake-sleep cycles are observed from fruit fly to human (Dunlap 1999). Though the reasons for sleeping may not yet been settled, given the need for sleeping, the reason for the circadian rhythms is fairly obvious, being dictated by the 24 h day-night cycle. Here we are concerned with why this rhythm is delayed for teenagers upon the onset of puberty. This delay is well-known by all parents with teenage children. It is very difficult to get adolescents to observe 'early to bed and early to rise'. It has also been clearly confirmed by scientific research, 'Our results indicate that pubertal maturation at this transitional phase (age 11–12 years) has a significant influence upon phase preference [i.e. delay in the circadian sleep cycle] and that psychosocial factors are less influential than anticipated' (Carskadon et al. 1993, p. 261; see also

---

[1] On the contribution of wisdom to the old, see Cheung and Chow (2020).

Gradisar et al. 2013). Thus, your teenage children' late sleeping habit is not mainly influenced by bad friends, but has a biological basis.

Why do teenagers sleep late? In biological research, there is a distinction between proximate versus ultimate reasons (Mayr 1961). The physiological mechanisms influencing the circadian rhythms and the differences of these factors for teenagers have been explored. A proximate reason for sleeping delay of teenagers is the delay in the secretion of melatonin in the body since puberty (Hagenauer et al. 2009; Troxel and Wolfson 2017). (Melatonin is related to sleeping. Thus, when one has jet lags, taking melatonin about 45 min before sleeping may help.) But why does this delay take place and at puberty? This more ultimate reason for this teenage delay in the rhythm has not, to my knowledge, been discussed. Here, I wish to advance a likely ultimate explanation.

The fact that the onset of the phase delay occurs at puberty suggests that it is related to mating. A person becomes potentially sexually active after puberty. Mating is directly related to the passing on of one's genes and hence takes priority over many other things (with the possible exception of survival). Thus, after puberty, allowing the individual to have high chance of mating becomes a high priority. Why is this related to the circadian phase delay?

The answer is hinted at in an ancient Chinese poem from the Song Dynasty: 'The moon rising up the top of the willow tree; people dating after nightfall' (Ouyang Xiu 欧阳修). Mating is more appropriate or common after nightfall. This is so both for privacy and safety, as one is more vulnerable to attack while mating. Thus, to have more opportunities for mating (and the pre-mating courting), adolescents have to delay sleeping time until well after nightfall. Given that it is probably easier and less harmful to delay than to shorten the sleeping time, the teenage circadian delay then emerged from mutation and got selected. This is our mating-facilitating explanation for the delay.

This delay helps partly explain the low happiness levels for both the teenagers and the middle aged. The belief in the desirability of 'early to bed and early to rise makes a person healthy, wealthy, and wise' is very deep-seated. Many schedules, including school and office hours observe this rule. When teenagers start to sleep and wake up late, they unavoidably get into conflict with their (mostly middle-aged) parents. This is likely one of the reasons accounting for the low happiness levels of these two groups.

Apart from having conflict with their parents, the delay in the sleep–wake cycles of teenagers also make them not having enough sleep, especially as the schooling hours have not been changed to fit their new biological clock (Carskadon et al. 2004). For the U.S., only about 7% of high-school students have enough sleep of 9 h a day needed for their ages (Basch et al. 2014). Evidence suggests no improvement in this and even some deterioration (Troxel and Wolfson 2017, p. 419).

One obvious social measure to tackle problems created by the delay in the teenagers' circadian cycle is to delay schooling hours for high schools. Why has this not been done. One reason is the inadequate recognition of this delay being biological rather than the influence of bad friends. Not realizing that this delay is natural tendency difficult to fight against makes people wanting the teenagers themselves to adjust to the social schedules.

Another reason against delaying hours for high schools is that this will increase transportation costs. Even if this is true, the benefits would likely be many times the costs. In fact, even if we confine only to the more easily measurable economic factors, the benefits are 9 times the costs (Jacob and Rockoff 2011). Even purely for productivity considerations, delaying high-school hours is highly desirable (Hafner et al. 2017).

Another reason against the delay in schooling hours for teenagers (high schools) is the argument that this delay will only delay further their hours of going to bed, not increasing the amount of their sleep. This is contradicted by a study showing that a delay of school hours by 50 min increases students' sleeping time by more than half an hour and reduces fatigue in day time (Owens et al. 2017). Some study concludes that delaying school start hours does not delay bedtime, but increases the amount of sleep, reduces daytime sleepiness, promote a better mood, and reduces coffee drinking (Boergers et al. 2014).

From many studies and experiments, it may be concluded that delaying schooling hours for teenagers not only increases their health, function, and safety, but also benefits the economy (Troxel and Wolfson 2017, p. 420). On the other hand, 'there was no evidence suggesting potential harmful outcomes associated with later start times for adolescents' (Troxel and Wolfson 2017, p. 421). Rather, inadequate sleep is obviously harmful, including affecting safety, as it will increase traffic accidents (Danner and Phillips 2008).

In April 2016, some southern districts of Maine in U.S. voted to delay secondary and high schools starting hours to no earlier than 8.30 (Collins et al. 2017). (Before this change, many schools started at around 7.30.) This decision affected 6,500 students. The delay in school starting hours produced positive effects, with no increase in transportation costs as afraid. People are now accustomed to the new hours. One personnel said, 'If you told our kids we'd be going back to the old system we'd have a revolt' (Collins et al. 2017, p. 482).

It seems clear that delaying starting hours for high schools is a simple way to increase sleeping time, health, and happiness for teenagers and their parents.

9.3 Chapter Appendix. Methodology

There are two different methods in analyzing the age-happiness relationship. The first is to directly look at the primary data, comparing the average happiness levels of individuals with different ages. This was used by early researchers, mainly psychologists. Within this method, there are also two different ways of analysis. The first is to compare the happiness levels of people of different age groups in any one time, i.e. taking a cross-section of people in the society at the same time/period. Another is to follow a group of people through their life or as they age. This is the time-series data (with the panel data on a specific group one being more reliable), in contrast to the cross-section data. This second way takes a long time to complete the study and hence is more costly and less frequently used.

In contrast to just looking at the primary data, another method is to do multiple regression on the primary data, either the cross-section or the panel one. Apart from separating people into different ages, we add other possible variables like sex, jobs, incomes, health conditions, etc. to get the relationships of age itself with happiness. The need for doing this multiple regression is based on the following rationale. For simplicity, suppose (not really true) that female (or the blue-collar workers) age-happiness relationship is mountain shape, while the male (while-collar workers) one is U shape. Then, if we do not distinguish the two groups and put them together, we may get the result that the age-happiness curve is horizontal, i.e. no relationship. But this hide the opposite and hence offsetting relationships of the two groups. Also, the middle age may be happier due to their higher incomes; if the income factor is deducted, there may be no different. Similarly, the aged may be less happy because of lower health; excluding the health factor, happiness may be unchanged.

However, it may also be argued that, the middle aged have higher incomes precisely because of their higher age (compared to the younger groups) that increases their experience and hence their incomes. So, this should not be deducted. Similarly, the aged may be less healthy precisely because of being older. So, this factor should also not be deducted. Thus, both the method using just primary data and the method using multiple regression have some advantages and some inadequacies. We may use both methods and compare the results. In recent years, researchers used both methods and still obtained the result that the age-happiness relationship is largely U shape. For example, Blanchflower and Oswald (2017) show that, out of seven data sets, if we just look at the primary data, we have the U shape relationship for 5 sets out of 7. Using multiple regression, we have the U shape result for all the 7 sets. Moreover, the U shape relationship is very large.

References

BASCH, C. E., BASCH, C. H., RUGGLES, K. V., & RAJAN, S. (2014). Prevalence of sleep duration on an average school night among 4 nationally representative successive samples of American high school students, 2007–2013. *Preventing Chronic Disease, 11*, E216.

BEJA, Edsel L. The U-shaped relationship between happiness and age: evidence using world values survey data. *Quality & Quantity*, 52.4 (2018): 1817–1829.

BLANCHFLOWER, David G. & OSWALD, Andrew J. (2008). Hypertension and happiness across nations. *Journal of Health Economics, 27*, 218–233.

BLANCHFLOWER, David G. & OSWALD, Andrew J. (2017). Do humans suffer a psychological low in Midlife? Two approaches (with and without controls) in seven data sets, IZA Discussion Papers, No. 10958, Institute of Labor Economics (IZA), Bonn. Available at: https://www.econstor.eu/bitstream/10419/170942/1/dp10958.pdf

BOERGERS, J., GABLE, C. J., & OWENS, J. A. (2014). Later school start time is associated with improved sleep and daytime functioning in adolescents. *Journal of Developmental & Behavioral Pediatrics, 35*(1), 11–17.

References

BURNS, R. A., MITCHELL, P., SHAW, J., & ANSTEY, K. (2014). Trajectories of terminal decline in the wellbeing of older women: The DYNOPTA project. *Psychology and Aging, 29*, 44–56.

BUTKOVIC, A., TOMAS, J., SPANIC, A. M. , et al. (2020). Emerging adults versus middle-aged adults: Do they differ in psychological needs, self-esteem and life satisfaction. *Journal of Happiness Studies, 21*, 779–798. https://doi.org/10.1007/s10902-019-00106-w

CARSKADON, M. A., ACEBO, C., & JENNI, O. G. (2004). Regulation of adolescent sleep: implications for behavior. *Annals of the New York Academy of Sciences, 1021*(1), 276–291. Retrived from: https://doi.org/10.1196/annals.1308.032.

CARSKADON, M. A.., VIEIRA, C. & ACEBO, C. (1993). Association between puberty and delayed phase preference. *Sleep, 16*(3), 258–262.

CHENG, Terence C., POWDTHAVEE, Nattavudh, & OSWALD, Andrew J. (2017). Longitudinal evidence for a midlife nadir in human well-being: Results from four data sets. *Economic Journal, 127*(599), 126–142.

CHEUNG, C. & CHOW, E. O. (2020). Contribution of Wisdom to Well-Being in Chinese Older Adults. *Applied Research Quality Life, 15*, 913–930. https://doi.org/10.1007/s11482-019-9712-x

COLLINS, T. A., INDORF, C., & KLAK, T. (2017). Creating regional consensus for starting school later: A physician-driven approach in southern Maine. *Sleep Health, 3*(6), 479–482.

DANNER, F., & PHILLIPS, B. (2008). Adolescent sleep, school start times, and teen motor vehicle crashes. *Journal of Clinical Sleep Medicine, 4*(06), 533–535.

DEATON, A. (2008). Income, health, and well-being around the world: Evidence from the Gallup World Poll. *Journal of Economic Perspectives, 22*, 53–72.

DUNLAP, Jay C. (1999). Molecular bases for circadian clocks. *Cell, 96*(2), 271–290.

FUKUDA, Kosei. (2013). A happiness study using age-period-cohort framework. *Journal of Happiness Studies, 14*(1), 135–153.

GERDTHAM, U. G., & JOHANNESSON, M. (2001). The relationship between happiness, health, and socio-economic factors: Results based on Swedish microdata. *The Journal of Socio-Economics, 30*(6), 553–557.

GONZÁLEZ-CARRASCO, M., CASAS, F., MALO, S., VIÑAS, F., & DINISMAN, T. (2017). Changes with age in subjective well-being through the adolescent years: Differences by gender. *Journal of Happiness Studies, 18*(1), 63–88.

GRADISAR, Michael, et al. (2013). The sleep and technology use of Americans: Findings from the National Sleep Foundation's 2011 Sleep in America Poll. *Journalof Clinical Sleep Medicine, 9*(12), 1291–1299.

GRAHAM, Carol, and Julia Ruiz POZUELO (2017) . Happiness, stress, and age: How the U curve varies across people and places. *Journal of Population Economics* 30.1 (2017): 225–264.

GRAHAM, Carol, ZHOU, S., & ZHANG, J. (2017). Happiness and health in China: The paradox of progress. *World development, 96*, 231–244.

HAFNER, M., STEPANEK, M., & TROXEL, W. M. (2017). The economic implications of later school start times in the United States. *Sleep Health, 3*(6), 451–457.

HAGENAUER, M. H., PERRYMAN, J. I., LEE, T. M., & CARSKADON, M. A. (2009). Adolescent changes in the homeostatic and circadian regulation of sleep. *Developmental Neuroscience, 31*(4), 276–284.

JACOB, B.A. & ROCKOFF, J.E. (2011). *Organizing Schools to Improve Student Achievement: Start Times, Grade Configurations, and Teachehhr Assignments*. The Hamilton Project, Brookings Institution.

LAAKSONEN, Seppo. (2018). A research note: Happiness by age is more complex than U-shaped. *Journal of Happiness Studies, 19*(2), 471–482.

MAYR, Ernst. (1961). Cause and effect in biology. *Science, 134*(3489), 1501–1506.

MROCZEK, D.K., & SPIRO, A. (2005). Change in life satisfaction during adulthood: Findings from the Veterans Affairs Normative Aging study. *Journal of Personality and Social Psychology, 88*, 189–202.

OWENS, J. A., DEARTH-WESLEY, T., HERMAN, A. N., OAKES, J. M., & WHITAKER, R. C. (2017). A quasi-experimental study of the impact of school start time changes on adolescent sleep. *Sleep Health, 3*(6), 437–443.

TROXEL, W. M. & WOLFSON, A. R. (2017). The intersection between sleep science and policy: Introduction to the special issue on school start times. *Sleep Health: Journal of the National Sleep Foundation, 3*(6), 419–422.

WEISS, A., KING, J.E., INOUE-MURAYAM, M., MATSUZAMA, T. & OSWALD, A.J. (2012). Evidence for a midlife crisis in great apes consistent with the U-shape in human well-being, *Proceedings of the National Academy of Scences U S A*, 109, 19949–19952. Retrieved from: https://www.weforum.org/agenda/2017/08/youll-probably-have-a-midlife-happiness-crisis-heres-why.

Open Access This chapter is licensed under the terms of the Creative Commons Attribution 4.0 International License (http://creativecommons.org/licenses/by/4.0/), which permits use, sharing, adaptation, distribution and reproduction in any medium or format, as long as you give appropriate credit to the original author(s) and the source, provide a link to the Creative Commons license and indicate if changes were made.

The images or other third party material in this chapter are included in the chapter's Creative Commons license, unless indicated otherwise in a credit line to the material. If material is not included in the chapter's Creative Commons license and your intended use is not permitted by statutory regulation or exceeds the permitted use, you will need to obtain permission directly from the copyright holder.

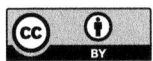

Chapter 10
Factors Affecting Happiness

Abstract Many factors may affect happiness, including how our needs (including the five levels identified by Maslow) are satisfied. Four important F's for happiness at the individual level are: faith, form/fitness, family, and friends. At the social level, important factors include environmental quality, equality, social capital (including trust).

10.1 Maslow's Hierarchy of Needs

We may look at our needs before examining factors affecting our happiness. A well-known list of needs is Maslow's (1943, 1954/1970a/1987) hierarchy of five levels/stages.[1] The first (most basic) level is the basic physiological needs of clothing, food, shelter, and sex. Next comes that of safety (including personal, employment and health); followed by love, friendship and belonging; and the fourth level of esteem, including achievement, being respected, and good reputation.[2] The highest fifth level is that of self-actualization. (Maslow estimated that only 2% of people reached this stage.)

I am in strong agreement with all the first four levels, but strongly disagree with self-actualization. First, I think that, except for the two points mentioned below, if a person has achieved the basic needs, safety, love, and esteem, she has largely actualized herself; there is no need for an extra level of self-actualization. This extra could create another Hitler that achieve self-actualization to the serious detriments of others. Secondly, the needs of the first four levels should be related to happiness of the individual concerned. Thirdly, I do want a higher fifth level, not of self-actualization, but 'beyond oneself'. Having achieved those in the first four levels, or even before

---

[1] These five levels/stages have been expanded to include cognitive and aesthetic needs (Maslow 1970) and transcendence needs (Maslow 1970). For empirical studies of different needs, see Tay and Diener (2011) and Rodríguez-Meirinhos et al. (2020); for a recent critical discussion, see McLeod (2020).

[2] On the role of self-esteem, especially in mediating the contribution of modesty to happiness, see Zheng and Wu (2020).

that, one should go beyond oneself to include the welfare of others, even including that of animals (on which see the final Chap. 16.

Partly based on our needs, we may also classify factors affecting our happiness into the subjective (i.e. one's own) and objective. Subjective factors include: nature (genes, pregnancy; though pregnancy may also be regarded as a form of nurture) and nurture (nourishment, education and influence of family, school, society), including physical, personality, intelligence, emotional quotient, etc. The objective factors include: family, school, work unit, friends, society, etc. The subjective and objective factors actually interact with each other as well as with personal choice and random factors. In this process, factors such as health, mental conditions, personal relationships, income/consumption/wealth, work, life, leisure activities, etc. are all important. One also experiences happiness and unhappiness, which in turns have feedbacks to those (especially subjective) factors. Then, over time, we have dynamic evolution of the various factors and happiness levels.

10.2 The Four F's of Happiness

Many years ago, I once (in public lectures) selected out of many factors for happiness, four particularly important ones for discussion. These are: Faith, Form/Fitness, Family, Friends—the four F's of happiness. Why four and not three or five. This is so because there is a well-known four F's in animal behavior. Except for sleeping (when hardly any behavior is involved), most if not all animals engage in the four F's most of the time: Feeding, Fighting, Fleeing, Mating. (Please do not ask me or anyone else: Why they are called the four F's, as the fourth one is an M, not an F?).

Faith includes in particular religious faith. Believers are happier than non-believers (Gundlachand Opfinger 2013). It may be that hope and spirituality may be more important here, rather than participation of religious rituals as such (Marques et al. 2013). I was brought up in a completely non-religious family. My father was a strong believer in materialism/communism in philosophy/politics; my mother, though believing in the existence of ghosts, did not practice any religious activities. However, influenced by my father, teachers, and the general atmosphere at the time (1950's in Malaya, the main constituent of Malaysia), I was a strong believer in communism as well. Since the second year in high school, I also actively participated in the communist-led student activities. Our faith and activities then actually also contributed much to our happiness then, though also likely to the miseries of some, including those expelled from schools, imprisoned, and even killed.

The importance of religious faith to happiness is likely underestimated. Religious belief is related negatively to incomes. Despite lower incomes, the believers are happier (Inglehart 2010). Thus, the positive effect of faith to happiness must be strong enough to offset the negative effect of incomes.

The factor of 'form/fitness' refers to health, including both physical and mental health. Though this factor has an important element of nature (what one is born with), nurture is also important. I can say this partly from my personal experience. I am the last (seventh) child in my family. Perhaps the factory of my mother's womb had been overworked by then (more than nine pregnancies including the still-born), I was born with somewhat below average health (and height). I remember having more illness including flu and toothache than most fellow school mates. I maintained frequent, though irregular exercises until I finished my first degree. After that, during my three years doing my PhD and the first few years as a lecturer, I had no serious exercise except mowing the lawn during spring/summer time after we bought our house. I reckon that over these 7 years or so of lack of exercise, my health conditions further deteriorated from its slightly below average level. Having realizing that, I started gradually to increase my exercise levels since around my mid 30's. Now, I am spending about 90 min virtually every day exercising; about an hour in the morning of breathing, stretching, standups, pushups, and gongfu, plus half an hour of taiji before going to bed. After decades of catching up, my health level is now far above people of the same age, and also above myself at my thirties.

Health is not just affected by nature and exercise, but also by one's attitude to life, lifestyle including healthy food and enough sleep. This is true for both physical and mental health.

I have a particular need to stay healthy and live long, at least until my 100 birthday in 2042. The story started from my teaching a Ford class (Sino-American Economics Training Centre) of graduates in Renmin University in Beijing over 1992–1993. Towards the end of that semester in March 1993, I made an appointment with the 40 students in the class to have a reunion after 16.5 years. Twenty of the forty students attended the reunion on 30 September 1999. At the end of the reunion, we made another appointment for another reunion after $16.5 \times 2 = 33$ years from then, or on 30 September 2042, when I will already be 100 years old. Since not many in that Ford class may be able to attend the next reunion, we also decided to extend the invitation to all my students. If you regard yourself as my student, you may come. Moreover, since I could do only about 20 pushups when I was in my 20 s, and 60 pushups in my 60 s, I will try to do 100 pushups in one go then. Thus, I have to live long and stay healthy. I am doing around 78 pushups every morning now, and adding one more every year. By 2042, I should be able to do 100! Haha!

For the last two F's of happiness: family and friends. I will say a few words on the last factor (friends) before discussing 'family' a little more later.

The importance of friendship for happiness is obvious for everyone. There are quite a few old Chinese sayings relating to this, e.g. 'At home, you rely on your parents; away from home, you rely on your friends'; 'With friends coming from afar, I am so happy!' In many Western countries, it is very important for many men to have a pint of bear with friends chatting at a bar. Studies also confirm the importance of friendship for happiness. However, it is more important to have one or a few good friends with whom one can share intimate joys and sorrows than having many friends. Here, it seems that quality is much more important than quantity.

The company of some friends enhances the mood at good activities and even turn negative moods into positive for undesirable activities. 'For example, to hike or walk alone raises mood by 2%, while a shared walk raises mood by much more, by 7.5% with a friend or 8.9% with a partner. Activities that normally worsen moods can induce happiness when done in the company of a friend or partner. Commuting or traveling, activities that on average worsen mood levels (−1.9%) are happiness-inducing when shared with friends or partners, with mood up 5.3% for a trip shared with a friend, or 3.9% with a partner. Even waiting or queueing, a significant negative when done alone (-3.5%) becomes a net positive when the experience is done with the company of a friend (+3.5%)' (World Happiness Report 2020, Chap. 1).[3]

Now on family. Before one forms one's own family, the relationship with parents and siblings are very important for happiness.[4] Similarly, these relationships are also very important for the happiness of parents. Most people have personal understanding of these from personal experience, if not also from watching TV and reading novels. When one grows up, one may get married to form one's own family. Despite the popular saying 'marriage is the grave of love', marriage is actually, on average, good for happiness.

In 2018, a study in U.S. lasting for three decades, discovered that 40% of the married regarded themselves as very happy; for those not married, this figure is only 24%. This is not a special case. Actually, many happiness studies consistently find that the married are happier than those not married. For happiness, marriage and employment are twice as important as incomes (Caroll 2007). Some researcher even estimated that, on average, a single person has to increase her/his income level to 13.8 times the existing level, to attain the same happiness level as the married (Dockery 2005).[5] Note that this is not 13.8% higher, but 13.8 times the original income. Except for very unusual fortunes, this huge increase in income is almost impossible; it is easier to get married. However, one must not marry any other person of the opposite sex. You have to find the right person. Those trying to get a divorce are much less happy than the singles. One aspect of a suitable spouse is similarity in personality (agreeableness and openness in particular) and values (moral identity and spirituality) which contribute not only to the life satisfaction of the couple but also the children (Wu et al. 2020).

You may suspect that the causal relationship may be reversed. It may not be that marriage increases your happiness; rather, it may be that the happier persons choose to marry, or easier to get a mate. While this reverse causal effect is likely applicable to some extent, further research shows that the beneficial effects of marriage on happiness are more important (Horiand Kamo 2017; Tao 2019).[6] Groverand Helliwell (2019, Abstract) 'control individual pre-marital well-being levels and find that the married are still more satisfied, suggesting a causal effect at all stages of the marriage, from pre-nuptual bliss to marriages of long-duration'.

---

[3] On the importance of engagement with family and friends for children happiness, see Savahl et al. (2020).

[4] On the importance of family, friends, and the school for children happiness, see Mínguez (2020); on the importance of parent–child relationship for the happiness of children, see Cherry et al. (2020).

[5] '... mean hourly earnings in 2002 were $A14.51. To have as great an impact on expected happiness as being married does for a a young male relative to being single would require earnings of in excess of $A200 per hour' (Dockery 2005, p. 300).

[6] Tao, focussing on Taiwan, in fact find no selection effect; married people were not happier 2 or more years before marriage. Also, 'Marriage, on average, enhances happiness more and longer for women' (Abstract).

10.2 The Four F's of Happiness

Why does marriage increase happiness? The most direct reason is the satisfaction of needs. Except for very few cases of artificial fertilization, sex between a man and a woman is needed to have babies and for the species to continue. Thus, to ensure the accomplishment of this mission, we have evolved the capacity for high enjoyment of sex.

You may argue that one does not have to get married to have sex. However, long-term well-adjusted partnership may achieve high levels in various relationships, not attainable by a one-night stand or commercial sex. In economic analysis, there is something called 'learning by doing'. This is also applicable to sexual relationship. Studies show that the best relationship is achieved after 15 years or longer: https://www.theguardian.com/lifeandstyle/2016/jul/23/why-sex-is-better-in-a-long-term-relationship.

About forty years ago, when the 50+ years old wife of a high official in China passed away, he was very sad. A colleague told him, 'With you wife gone, you may marry a younger one, isn't this nice?' When reading this report then, I was agreeable with that colleague. Now I understand more why that official was very sad. Though younger women are more attractive in look, a well-adjusted long-term partner is more beneficial to happiness, as studies show. Of course, apart from sex, there are also other relationships between a husband and wife. Man is a social animal and are born not to like loneliness.

From an economic or financial aspect, marriage is also advantageous. The ideas of division of labor and economies of scale also apply here. Men and women are good in different things and can cooperate to achieve much better results in many areas. Cooking for two persons certainly costs much less than twice the time of doing that for one person.

A few years back, an interesting paper entitled 'Are all good men married? The conclusion is: 'Not that all good men are married; but rather, after being married and having a good wife to assist him, that he becomes a high-earning good man' (王智波、李长洪 2016, 第838页; my translation) . Thus, with the right partner, marriage is likely an arrangement that is most mutually beneficial.

Since marriage is good for us financially, biologically, and spiritually, why is the institution of marriage seems to be on the decline, with some people (e.g. 俞炜华 2011) even regarding it as being restrictive of human nature and will vanish in due course? (See 黄有光 2013 for a defense of the institution of marriage against this argument.)

First, though marriage is good for our happiness, many do not sufficiently recognize this fact. For example, in Netherlands and the U.S., most people believe that marriage will not increase our life satisfaction, but actually, studies show that their life satisfaction is positively affected by marriage (Kapteyn et al. 2010, p. 99).

Secondly, we are usually misled by news reports and gossips. We often hear that someone's marriage has broken up, or the relationship is in trouble, making people believe that 'marriage is the grave of love'. Actually, most happy marriages attract little reports and gossips, but marriages in trouble do. When you enjoy yourself much in your home, you do not talk to friends and relatives about it; when you have relationship problems, you may seek help from them. This asymmetry may mislead bystanders. This is related to the saying, 'Good news does not go out of your doorstep; bad news is spread thousands of miles away'.

One example of the exaggeration of bad news is this. Over many decades, it has been said that more than 50% of marriages in the U.S. will end up in divorce, and that this figure is still increasing. Actually, this was only an estimated figure for the future that never realizes. In the 1970's, after the relaxation of the divorce laws in the U.S., the rates of divorce increased rapidly. Someone then extrapolated the future divorce rates to break the 50% line, based on that short-term increase. But this prediction never comes true. Actually, the divorce rates in the U.S. have declined substantially over the last four decades, with the number of divorces for every thousand married women declining from 22.6 in 1980 to 16.9 in 2015, and remaining around this lower figure since. However, the 50% figure has spread widely and still believed by many.

Yet another reason for the underestimation of the benefits of marriage is that these benefits are largely longer-term, not fully realized in the short run. According to a U.S. study (Amatoand James 2018), happiness increases after marriage, but then decreases somewhat over the next few years, reaching a low at around 5–10 years after marriage. Thus, the so-called 'seven-years itch' has some validity. Nevertheless, after more than ten or twenty years after marriage, happiness increases back significantly. A report by the government of Shanghai shows a similar result. More than 80% of women in Shanghai are happy, but those women married for less than three years have the lowest happiness levels. Those with the highest happiness levels have been married for 20 years or longer, as reported in United Morning Daily, Singapore's leading Chinese newspaper (《联合早报》2015.10.28). Marriage has to be cultivated for a long time to produce great happiness.

Thus, the saying 'Marriage is the grave of love' is largely based on unreliable guess, inaccurate or misleading reports/gossips, and the inadequate recognition of the long-term effects. Thus, persons of marriageable age should not be misled by this saying. They should get a good partner to marry.

In 2014, at a function for new students, I was asked to give a talk. Among other points, I mentioned this. During this few years of study, do not just get a degree; get a partner as well. University study is the golden age for finding a partner: more opportunities, more information, more sincerity. However, I also told them, 'If you have not got a partner yet, you cannot beat me, because my wife and I started dating each other in our high school days and got married soon after our degrees!'.

For those already married, they should not give it up easily. It may take time to make a marriage work well. However, for those unsalvageable relationship, the divorce option should not be excluded altogether. Instead of suffer a long time to maintain an unhappy marriage, ending the relationship and get a new start may be better.

These days, many people cohabitate without getting married. Is cohabitation as good as marriage for happiness? A study in the U.K. shows that both cohabitation and happiness are good for happiness. However, for those first time getting married, marriage increases life satisfaction more than cohabitation does (Blekesaune 2018).

For people in the East, due to the higher traditional views about marriage, this advantage of marriage over cohabitation is likely to be even bigger. Also, a higher degree of commitment in partnership increases life satisfaction (Bucher et al. 2019).

There is an interesting difference between men and women regarding marriage. A study on more than two thousand persons (Liu et al. 2013) shows that, for men's life satisfaction, whether one is married or not is important; for women, the quality of the marriage is more important. The old Chinese saying, 'It is important for a man not to enter a wrong business; it is important for a woman not to marry a wrong husband', has some validity. Of course, the quality of marriage is important for both men and women; however, it is more important for women. Thus, the extra care (in comparison to men) taken by a woman in choosing a partner does not only have an evolutionary reason (Sect. 10.3), but also a rational one (consistent with happiness calculation).

There is another interesting finding in China. For those university-educated females, those with the highest happiness level are 'with family but no job'; next comes those 'with family and job'; further down are those with 'job but no family'. The least happy are those with neither job nor family (吴要武、刘倩 2014, 第27页). Family and job are both important, but at least for females, family is more important than job.

An important question especially for parents is: For the future happiness when grown up, what factors are important when young? Layard et al. (2014) show that the most important factor is emotional health, followed by characters or conduct, with the least important one being intellectual development, out of these three important factors. Thus, for the true happiness of children rather than your own face, do not give too much pressure on children to perform well in examination; much more important to help them develop well on emotional health, and behave properly, particularly by setting examples yourselves.

10.3 Important Factors at the Social Level

The above factors affecting happiness, the 4 F's in particular, focus at the individual level. For the social level, there are many other factors important for the happiness of individuals in the society. This include environmental quality, equality (in the distribution of incomes and wealth), freedom, democracy, government quality (Helliwelland Huang 2008), social capital, etc. On the importance of social capital, see Neira et al. 2019; on the importance of trust, an important element of social capital, see Hudson 2006; Helliwelland Wang 2011; Helliwell et al. 2014; on the importance of social trust especially for urban males, see Lu et al. 2020, b; on the importance of mental capital, which is more on the individual level, see Ho 2013. Also, Chap. 7 of the World Happiness Report 2020 finds that higher personal and institutional trust are key factors in explaining why life evaluations are high in the Nordic countries.

On democracy, Frey and Stutzer (2002) comparing situations in different cantons in Switzerland, find that direct election is positively associated with happiness, both in getting people's preferred results, and also in higher satisfaction in the democratic process. On the other hand, Chinese researchers (陈前恒 et al. 2014) find that each 1% increase in democratic development in the village, increases well-being equivalent to 18.47% increase in per-capita net income. This is a huge effect. (On the importance of political participation on farmers' happiness, see also Tang et al. 2020.)

Freedom is positively associated with happiness (Veenhoven 2000), but mainly for rich countries; not for poor countries, except for economic freedom. Free trade related positively to happiness in poor, but not in rich countries. This is consistent with the higher positive relationship of income levels before US$7,500 per-capita per year than after this level. Free trade increases effective consumption and hence is important for people at lower incomes. Similarly, economic and legal institutions are more important to low-income countries, while political institutions are more important to rich countries (Bjornskov et al. 2010; Helliwell et al. 2014). On the importance of economic freedom, see also Graafland (2020) especially on the interdependence of culture and institutions.

Equality (in both income and wealth distribution) increases happiness in many ways. First, human beings are not as strong as tigers physically, and hence we rely largely on our intelligence (in its generalized sense of including IQ, EQ and wisdom) and cooperation to survive and prosper. Our sense for equality and justice helps us to cooperate better and hence we are probably universally born with a preference for equality. This is further strengthened by nurture as our education and culture are also equality-friendly. Hence, a higher degree of equality, if not achieved at prohibitive costs, allows the society to be better off because individuals directly feel better off with higher equality.

Secondly, consumption of the poor meets more urgent needs than that of the rich, at the margin. That is to say, the last one thousand dollars of spending probably contribute little if anything to the utility or welfare of a rich person, but may mean a lot to one with low consumption. Thus, a higher degree of equality promotes more aggregate welfare, through the differentials in the marginal utility of consumption. This argument is based on the interpersonal comparability of cardinal utility/welfare that many economists frown upon traditionally, but is defended in Chap. 6 above. The age of insisting upon only ordinal measurability and interpersonal non-comparability is, or at least should be, over.

Thirdly, equality reduces crimes and promotes social harmony. This has been known for a long time. However, recent research emphasizing the efficiency-promoting effects of equality has shifted economists' view. Formerly, economists (e.g. Mirrlees 1971; Okun 1975/2015) focused on the tradeoff between equality and efficiency. That is, if we promote equality, we need to sacrifice a bit of efficiency, e.g. taxing the rich to help the poor incurs not only administrative costs, but also creates the disincentive effects that discourage the earning of more money. Now, economists focus on the beneficial effects of equality on efficiency and growth.

One important aspect here is related to the shift from physical to human capital as being important for economic growth. When physical capital was important, inequality increased growth by increasing savings by the rich and hence increased capital accumulation and economic growth; as human capital becomes more important, equality increases the contribution of widespread education and hence growth (Milanovic 2011). In addition, 'Economic historians have shown (Solar 1995; Greifand Iyigun 2013) that the net effect of the Poor Law was probably to foster technological progress, because it weakened the resolve of the inevitable losers to resist it and thus reduced social unrest' (Mokyr 2014, p.192). Also, '…economic historians such as Lindert (2004, 2009) … have shown the complex, but on the whole favorable, effect of the Welfare State on economic performance to the point where the full economic benefits and costs may have been roughly equal, making the Welfare State a "free lunch"' (Mokyr 2014, p.191). This suggests that more equality-improving welfare spending may be welfare improving, since equality also contributes to welfare more directly as discussed above.[7] This is consistent with a recent result that 'Tax policy that alleviates poverty improves economic growth in most instances' (Biswas et al. 2017, p. 724).

Equality also reduces crimes and increases social harmony and trust, and trust increases happiness (Uslaner 2001). There is much evidence that inequality is negative to happiness; see Hagerty (2000), Fahey and Smyth (2004), Oshioand Urakawa (2013), Huang et al. (2016), Ding et al. (2020) and the second half of Chap. 2, World Happiness Report 2020. Oishi et al. (2012) show that countries with higher progressivity in the income tax system have higher happiness levels. Using data in China, Ding et al. (2020, Abstract) show that 'both absolute and relative income affect subject well-being, and that an inverted-U shaped relationship between income inequality and individual well-being appears at least for urban residents, whereas this relationship tend to be negative in the case of people living in rural areas'. There are also indirect evidence of the desirability of equality. In the U.S., regional death rates are highly related to inequality (Kaplan et al. 1996; Lynch et al. 1998). In Italy, inequality is more important than income and education for the effects on death rates (De Vogli et al. 2005).[8]

The importance of equality is not only for its material/financial aspects, but for the sense of justice/fairness. (On the negative effects of inequality in both income and life satisfaction on trust and hence happiness, see Graaflandand Lous 2019.) A small story may be told here. Decades ago in China under Mao, dating at high school was much discouraged if not outright prohibited. A young couple disobeyed the advice not to date. Partly as a means to separate the two, the boy was sent down to the village. Though not sent down to the much difficult living and working conditions of a village, the girl went to stay with her lover in the village. Then came the Autumn Festival and each family was distributed with one mooncake. The youngster came home with the mooncake before his lover came home. During those days of starvation, he

---

[7] For studies showing some efficiency-enhancing features of equality, see also references cited at the end of Chap. 6 of Ng 2000.

[8] However, see Hirschmanand Rothschild (1973) and Davis (2019) on the tunnel effect or 'the propensity for individuals to be pleased by the success of others if they believe this signals an improvement in their own prospects'. Also, on the importance of perceived (instead of actual) inequality, see Schalembier (2019).

could not resist the temptation of eating half of the cake before her return. However, once tasting the delicious mooncake in a semi-hunger situation, he could not restrain himself and ended up swallowing the whole cake. When the girl came back, she happily asked, 'I heard that we have a mooncake'. He sadly told her that he had eaten it all. She kept silent for a few minutes, and then burst out, 'I follow you to the horrible conditions of the village to be with you. And ... And you did not even keep my share of the cake for me?!' She packed up and left him to go back home to the city. What the strong state power failed to separate was easily done by half a mooncake.

An issue related to inequality is relative income/consumption/standing. In economics, this has been analysed from Rae (1834) and Veblen (1899) to Frank (1999). This relative competition is not just important for the rich; even in poor villages in China and India, it is more important than absolute income (Luttmer 2005; Knight et al. 2009a, b; Knightand Gunatilaka 2010; Linssen et al. 2011; Guillen-Royo 2011; Fontaineand Yamada 2012. Cf. Garrard 2012; Huang et al. 2016; Li 2017; Asadullah et al. 2018; Luo et al. 2018; Collischon 2019; Sherman et al. 2019; Bakkeli 2020; Zhangand Wang, 2020). Some researchers (e.g. Layard et al. 2010) even regard 'All effects are relative'. This resonates with the Confucian saying that 'No worry about poverty, but about inequality'. Even in health care, where one expects that the absolute levels are more important, relative standing is more important than absolute level. The relatively poor, even with higher absolute income and health care, have lower absolute health outcomes (Wilkinson 1997).

The importance of relative standing is largely evolutionary-biological. To pass on your genes you need to attract good mates. Here, it is more important to be better than your competitors than just to have high values. This is particularly so for males. Before the short history of common monogamy, the head-man of a tribe could mate with all women. But a woman is limited by the requirement of 9 months of pregnancy, years of nursing and caring to ensure that the child will be able to survive. Thus, men are more competitive, trying to go to the top, much more than women. However, that they have the higher urge does not necessarily means that they are also better leaders than women. With their higher EQ and language abilities, perhaps women are better leaders.

I mentioned this during a class of a dozen PhD students at Monash University more than ten years ago. A female student from China objected that a woman should only be No. 2, not No.1. I was very surprised and asked why. She said that women are more emotional, especially during their monthly periods. Perhaps she had a point. But an Australian girl student objected very vehemently. The Chinese girl said, 'See! Aren't you very emotional now?' When I told this story to another class at Nanyang Technological University some years later, a male student said that, by the time she is ready to lead either a nation, an enterprise, or a university, a woman is typically well pass the time of having monthly periods. This is largely true. However, the Chinese girl student may still be right that, even outside the monthly periods, women are more emotional. Also, the recent birth of a baby by the young female prime minister of New Zealand is also a counter example. Likely a counter example in both the following opposite senses: that they are no longer having periods; that they are too emotional to lead well. As often, many factors are involved.

There is another troubling gender difference. In early decades of happiness study, at least in the U.S., women happiness was originally found to be higher than men. However, in recent decades, despite (or because of ?) much higher gender equalization, this advantage of women has decreased and disappeared (Kahneman et al. 1999; Stevensonand Wolfers 2009).[9] Kahneman believes that this may be due to more honesty in report or higher demands due to higher opportunities. Thus, this is related to the possible divergences between true happiness and reported happiness. Ho (2013) disagrees and believes that it may be due to the higher housework responsibilities of women, despite both having full-time jobs. Also, Audette et al. (2019) find the promotion of gender equality increases happiness for both sexes. Again, multiple factors are likely involved and further studies are needed.

Employment and price stability are also important for happiness. In economics, there is a well-known formula that the misery index = unemployment rate + inflation rate. However, according to happiness studies, this formula should be seriously revised. Instead of being equally important in contributing to happiness or misery, each percentage point of unemployment reduces happiness 5 times that of each percentage point of inflation (Blanchflower et al. 2014). It is interesting to note that an increase in unemployment benefits increases the happiness of both the unemployed and the employed (Di Tella et al. 2003). With reasonable unemployment benefits, perhaps the employed also feel more secure. Also, while people may adjust or adapt, over time, to many problems, but it is very difficult to adjust to being unemployed, even given time (Clark and Georgellis 2013).

References

AMATO, P. R., & JAMES, S. L. (2018). Changes in spousal relationships over the marital life course,In: Alwin D., Felmlee D., Kreager D. (eds). *Social Networks and the Life Course*, Frontiers in Sociology and Social Research, vol 2. Springer, Cham, pp. 139–158. Available at: https://www.businessinsider.sg/happiest-point-in-marriage-2018-4/?r=US&IR=T.

ASADULLAH, M. N., XIAO, S., & YEOH, E. (2018). Subjective well-being in China, 2005–2010: The role of relative income, gender, and location. *China Economic Review, 48*, 83–101.

AUDETTE, A. P., LAM, S., O'CONNOR, H. et al. (2019). Quality of Life: A Cross-National Analysis of the Effect of Gender Equality on Life Satisfaction. *Journal of Happiness Studies, 20*(7), 2173–2188. https://doi.org/10.1007/s10902-018-0042-8.

BAKKELI, N. Z. (2020). Older adults' mental health in China: Examining the relationship between income inequality and subjective wellbeing using panel data Analysis. *Journal of Happiness Studies, 21*(4), 1349–1383. https://doi.org/10.1007/s10902-019-00130-w.

BISWAS, Siddhartha, CHAKRABORTY, Indraneel, & HAI, Rong. (2017). Income inequality, tax policy, and economic growth. *Economic Journal, 127*(601), 688–727.

---

[9] Also, 'Black women … present a consistent pattern of improvement in happiness across decades, while White women display a persistent pattern of decline' (Cummings 2020, Abstract). Relevant factors are likely complex.

BJORNSKOV, Christian, DREHER, Axel & FISCHER, Justina A. V. (2010). Formal institutions and subjective well-being: Revisiting the cross-country evidence. *European Journal of Political Economy, 26*(4), 419–430.

BLANCHFLOWER, D., BELL, David N. F., MONTAGNOLI, A. & MORO, M. (2014). The happiness tradeoff between unemployment and inflation. *Journal of Money, Credit and Banking, 46*(S2), 117–141.

BLEKESAUNE, Morten. (2018). Is cohabitation as good as marriage for people's subjective well-being? Longitudinal evidence on happiness and life satisfaction in the British household panel survey. *Journal of Happiness Studies, 19*(2), 505–520.

BUCHER, A., NEUBAUER, A.B., VOSS, A. , et al. (2019). Together is better: Higher committed relationships increase life satisfaction and reduce loneliness. *Journal of Happiness Studies, 20,* 2445–2469. https://doi.org/10.1007/s10902-018-0057-1.

CARROLL, Nick. (2007). Unemployment and psychological well-being. *Economic Record, 83*(262), 287–302.

CHERRY, K. M., MCARTHUR, B. A., & LUMLEY, M. N. (2020). A Multi-Informant Study of Strengths, Positive Self-Schemas and Subjective Well-Being from Childhood to Adolescence. *Journal of Happiness Studies, 21,* 2169–2191. https://doi.org/10.1007/s10902-019-00171-1.

CLARK, A. E., & GEORGELLIS, Y. (2013). Back to baseline in Britain: Adaptation in the British Household Panel Survey. *Economica, 80*(319), 496–512.

COLLISCHON, Matthias. (2019). Relative pay, rank and happiness: A comparison between genders and part-and full-time employees. *Journal of Happiness Studies, 20*(1), 67–80.

CUMMINGS, J. L. (2020). Assessing U.S. Racial and Gender Differences in Happiness, 1972–2016: An Intersectional Approach. Journal of Happiness Studies 21(2): 709–735. https://doi.org/10.1007/s10902-019-00103-z.

DAVIS, L. (2019). Growth, Inequality and Tunnel Effects: A Formal Mode. *Journal of Happiness Studies, 20,* 1103–1119. https://doi.org/10.1007/s10902-018-9991-1.

DE VOGLI, R., MISTRY, R., GNESOTTO, R., & CORNIA, G. A. (2005). Has the relation between income inequality and life expectancy disappeared? Evidence from Italy and top industrialised countries. *Journal of Epidemiology and Community Health, 59,* 158–162.

DI TELLA, R., MACCULLOCH, R., & OSWALD, A. (2003). The Macroeconomics of Happiness. *Review of Economics and Statistics, 85*(4), 809–827.

DING, J., SALINAS-JIMÉNEZ, J., & SALINAS-JIMÉNEZ, M.d. (2020). The impact of income inequality on subjective well-being: The case of China. *Journal of Happiness Studies.* https://doi.org/10.1007/s10902-020-00254-4.

DOCKERY, A. M. (2005). The happiness of young Australians: Empirical evidence on the role of labour market experience. *Economic Record, 81*(255), 322–335.

FAHEY, T., & SMYTH, E. (2004). Do subjective indicators measure welfare? Evidence from 33 European societies. *European Societies, 6,* 5–27.

FONTAINE, Xavier & YAMADA, Katsunori (2012). Economic comparison and group identity: Lessons from India, hal-00711212, version 2.

FRANK, R. H. (1999). *Luxury Fever: Why Money Fails to Satisfy in an Era of Excess.* Free Press.

FREY, Bruno S. & STUTZER, Alois. (2002). *Happiness and Economics: How the Economy and Institutions Affect Well-Being.* Princeton University Press.

GARRARD, Graeme. (2012). The status of happiness. *International Review of Economics, 59*(4), 377–387.

GRAAFLAND, J., & LOUS, B. (2019). Income Inequality, Life Satisfaction Inequality and Trust: A Cross Country Panel Analysis. *Journal of Happiness Studies, 20,* 1717–1737. https://doi.org/10.1007/s10902-018-0021-0

GRAAFLAND, J. (2020). When Does Economic Freedom Promote Well Being? On the Moderating Role of Long-Term Orientation. *Social Indicators Research, 149,* 127–153. https://doi.org/10.1007/s11205-019-02230-9.

GREIF, Avner & IYIGUN, Murat (2013). What did the old poor law really accomplish? Aredux. Institute for the Study of Labor Discussion Paper 7398.

References

GROVER, Shawn & John F. HELLIWELL. (2019). How's life at home? New evidence on marriage and the set point for happiness. *Journal of Happiness Studies, 20*(2), 373–390. https://doi.org/10.1007/s10902-017-9941-3.

GUILLEN-ROYO, Monica (2011). Reference group consumption and the subjective wellbeing of the poor in Peru. *Journal of Economic Psychology*, 259–272.

GUNDLACH, E., & OPFINGER, M. (2013). Religiosity as a determinant of happiness. *Review of Development Economics, 17*(3), 523–539.

HAGERTY, M. R. (2000). Social comparisons of income in one's community: Surveys of income and happiness. *Journal of Personality and Social Psychology, 78*, 746–771.

HELLIWELL, J., & HUANG, H. (2008). How's Your Government? International Evidence Linking Good government and Well-being. *British Journal of Political Science, 38*, 595–619.

HELLIWELL, John F., HUANG, Haifang, & WANG, Shun. (2014). Social capital and well-being in times of crisis. *Journal of Happiness Studies, 15*, 145–162.

HELLIWELL, John F., WANG, Shun. (2011). Trust and well-being. *International Journal of Wellbeing, 1*(1), 42–78.

HIRSCHMAN, A. O., & ROTHSCHILD, M. (1973). The changing tolerance for income inequality in the course of economic development: With a mathematical appendix. *The Quarterly Journal of Economics, 87*(4), 544–566.

HO, Lok Sang. (2013). *The Psychology and Economics of Happiness: Love, Life and Positive Living*. Routledge.

HORI, Makiko and KAMO, Yoshinori (2017). Gender differences in happiness: The effects of marriage, social roles, and social support in East Asia. Applied Research in Quality of Life, 1–19. DOI: https://doi.org/10.1007/s11482-017-9559-y.

HUANG, J., WU, S., & DENG, S. (2016). Relative income, relative assets, and happiness in urban China. *Social Indicators Research, 126*(3), 971–985.

HUDSON, J. (2006). Institutional trust and subjective well-being across the EU. *Kyklos, 59*(1), 43–62.

INGLEHART, Ronald F. (2010). Faith and freedom traditional and modern ways to happiness, in Diener et al, pp. 351–397.

KAHNEMAN, Daniel, DIENER, Ed & SCHWARZ, Norbert, (Ed.). (1999). *Well-Being: The Foundations of Hedonic Psychology*. Russell Sage Foundation.

KAPLAN, G. A., PAMUK, E. R., LYNCH, J. W., COHEN, R. D. & BALFOUR, J. L. (1996). Inequality in income and mortality in the United States: Analysis of mortality and potential pathways. *British Medical Journal, 312*, 999–1003.

KAPTEYN, Arie, SMITH, James P. & VAN SOEST, Arthur (2010). *Life Satisfaction*, In Diener et al., pp. 70–104.

KNIGHT, John & GUNATILAKA, Ramani. (2010). Great expectations? *The Subjective Well-Being of Rural-Urban Migrants in China, World Development, 38*(1), 113–124.

KNIGHT, John, SONG, Lina & GUNATILAKA, Ramani (2009a). Subjective well-being and its determinants in rural China. *China Economic Review*, 20(4): 635–649.

KNIGHT, John, SONG, Lina & GUNATILAKA, Ramani (2009b). Subjective well-being and its determinants in rural China. *China Economic Review*, 20(4): 635–49.

LAYARD, R., MAYRAZ, G. & NICKELL, S. (2010). Does relative income matter? Are the critics right? In Diener, et al., pp. 139–165.

LAYARD, Richard, CLARK, Andrew E., CORNAGLIA, Francesca, POWDTHAVEE, Nattavudh, VERNOIT, Jame. What Predicts a Successful Life? A Life-Course Model of Well-Being. *The Economic Journal*, Volume 124, Issue 580, November 2014, Pages F720–F738, https://doi.org/10.1111/ecoj.12170.

LI, Weisen (2017). Self preface to The True Logic of China's Economic Growth. *China-Review Weekly* [《中评周刊》], 29: 7–11.

LINDERT, Peter H. (2004). *Growing Public: Volume 1, The Story: Social Spending and Economic Growth since the Eighteenth Century*. Cambridge and New York: Cambridge University Press.

LINDERT, Peter H. (2009). *Growing Public: Volume 2, Further Evidence: Social Spending and Economic Growth since the Eighteenth Century*. Cambridge and New York: Cambridge University Press.

LINSSEN, Rik, VAN KEMPEN, Luuk & KRAAYKAMP, Gerbert. (2011). Subjective well-being in rural India: The curse of conspicuous consumption. *Social Indicators Research, 101*(1), 57–72. https://doi.org/10.1007/s11205-010-9635-2.

LIU, H., LI, S., & FELDMAN, M.W. (2013). Gender in marriage and life satisfaction under gender imbalance in China: The role of intergenerational support and SES. *Social Indicators Research, 114*(3), 915–933.

LU, C., JIANG, Y., ZHAO, X. et al. (2020a). Will helping others also benefit you? Chinese adolescents' altruistic personality traits and life satisfaction. *Journal of Happiness Studies, 21*(4), 1407–1425. https://doi.org/10.1007/s10902-019-00134-6.

LU, H., TONG, P. & ZHU, R. (2020b). Longitudinal evidence on social trust and happiness in China: Causal effects and mechanisms. *Journal of Happiness Studies* 21, 1841–1858. DOI:https://doi.org/10.1007.

LUO, Yangmei, WANG, Tong, and HUANG, Xiting. (2018). Which types of income matter most for well-being in China: Absolute, relative or income aspirations? *International Journal of Psychology, 53*(3), 218–222.

LUTTMER, Erzo F. (2005). Neighbors as negatives: Relative earnings and well-being. *Quarterly Journal of Economics, 120*(3), 963–1002.

LYNCH, J., KAPLAN, G. A., PAMUK, E. R., COHEN, R. D., HECK, K. H., BALFOUR, J. L. & YEN, I. H. (1998). Income inequality and mortality in metropolitan areas of United States. *American Journal of Public Health, 88*, 1074–1080.

MARQUES, S., LOPEZ, S. & MITCHEll, J. (2013). The role of hope, spirituality and religious practice in adolescents' life satisfaction: Longitudinal findings. *Journal of Happiness Studies, 14*(1), 251–261.

MASLOW, A. H. (1943). A theory of human motivation. *Psychological Review, 50*(4), 370–396.

MASLOW, A. H. (1970). *Religions, Values, and Peak Experiences*. Penguin.

MASLOW, A. H. (1954/1970a/1987). *Motivation and Personality*. New York: Harper & Row/ Delhi, India: Pearson Education.

MCLEOD, S. A. (2020). *Maslow's Hierarchy of Needs*. Simply Psychology. https://www.simplypsychology.org/maslow.html.

MILANOVIC, Branko. (2011). More or less. *Finance & Development, 48*(3), 6–11.

MÍNGUEZ, A. M. (2020). Children's relationships and happiness: The role of family, friends and the school in four European countries. *Journal of Happiness Studies, 21*(5), 1859–1878. https://doi.org/10.1007/s10902-019-00160-4.

MIRRLEES, James A. (1971). An exploration in the theory of optimum income taxation. *Review of Economic Studies, 38*, 175–208.

MOKYR, J. (2014). A flourishing economist. *Journal of Economic Literature, 52*(1), 189–196.

NEIRA, I., LACALLE-CALDERON, M., PORTELA, M. et al. (2019). Social capital dimensions and subjective well-being: A quantile approach. *Journal of Happiness Studies, 20*, 2551–2579. https://doi.org/10.1007/s10902-018-0028-6.

NG, Yew-Kwang. (2000). *Efficiency, Equality, and Public Policy: With a Case for Higher Public Spending*. Macmillan.

OISHI, S., SCHIMMACK, U., and DIENER, E. (2012). Progressive taxation and the subjective well-being of nations. *Psychological Science, 23*(1), 86–92.

OKUN, Arthur M. (1975/2015), *Equality and Efficiency: The Big Tradeoff*, Washington: Brookings Institution.

RAE, John (1834). *New Principles of Political Economy*. Reprinted as *The Sociological Theory of Capital: Being a Complete Reprint of the News Principles of Political Economy*, 1905, The Macmillan Company.

RODRÍGUEZ-MEIRINHOS, A., ANTOLÍN-SUÁREZ, L., BRENNING, K. et al. (2020). A bright and a dark path to adolescents' functioning: The role of need satisfaction and need frustration across gender, age, and socioeconomic Status. *Journal of Happiness Studies, 21*, 95–116. https://doi.org/10.1007/s10902-018-00072-9.

SAVAHL, S., ADAMS, S., FLORENCE, M. et al. (2020). The relation between children's participation in daily activities, their engagement with family and friends, and subjective well-being. *Child Indicators Research, 13*, 1283–1312. https://doi.org/10.1007/s12187-019-09699-3.

SCHALEMBIER, B. (2019). An evaluation of common explanations for the impact of income inequality on life satisfaction. *Journal of Happiness Studies, 20*(3), 777–794. https://doi.org/10.1007/s10902-018-9970-6.

SOLAR, Peter. (1995). Poor relief and English economic development before the industrial revolution. *Economic History Review, 48*(1), 1–22.

STEVENSON, Betsey & WOLFERS, Justin. (2009). The Paradox of declining female happiness. *American Economic Journal: Economic Policy, 1*(2), 190–225.

TANG, L., LUO, X., YU, W. et al. (2020). The effect of political participation and village support on farmers happiness. *Journal of Chinese Political Science*. https://doi.org/10.1007/s11366-020-09680-w.

TAO, Hung-Lin. (2019). Marriage and happiness: Evidence from Taiwan. *Journal of Happiness Studies, 20*(6), 1843–1861. https://doi.org/10.1007/s10902-018-0029-5.

TAY, L. & DIENER, E. (2011). Needs and subjective well-being around the world. *Journal of Personality and Social Psychology, 101*(2), 354–356.

USLANER, E. (2001). *The Moral Foundations of Trust*. Cambridge University Press.

VEBLEN, T. (1899). *The Theory of the Leisure Class*. Macmillan.

VEENHOVEN, Ruut (2000). Freedom and happiness: A comparative study in 44 nations in the early 1990's. In DIENER E, SUH EM (eds), *Culture and Subjective Well-Being*, The MIT Press, Cambridge, MA, US, pp. 257–288.

WILKINSON, R. G. (1997). Health inequalities: Relative or absolute material standards? *British Medical Journal, 314*(22), 591–595.

World Happiness Report (2016, 2018, 2019, 2020, 2021). Retrieved from: https://worldhappiness.report/ed/2021/.

WU, R., LIU, Z., GUO, Q. et al. (2020). Couple similarity on personality, moral identity and spirituality predict life satisfaction of spouses and their offspring. *Journal of Happiness Studies, 21*, 1037–1058. https://doi.org/10.1007/s10902-019-00108-8.

ZHANG, Z. & WANG, X. (2020). Ambition or jealousy? It depends on whom you are compared with. *Journal of Happiness Studies*. DOI: https://doi.org/10.1007/s10902-020-00269-x.

ZHENG, C. & WU, Y. (2020). The more modest you are, the happier you are: The mediating roles of emotional intelligence and self-esteem. *Journal of Happiness Studies, 21*(5), 1603–1615. https://doi.org/10.1007/s10902-019-00144-4.

俞炜华 (2011)。《婚恋与选择》, 山东人民出版社。

吴要武、刘倩 (2014). 高校扩招对婚姻市场的影响: 剩女?剩男?《经济学季刊》, 14 (1) : 5–30.

王智波、李长洪 (2016). 好男人都结婚了吗?《经济学季刊》, 15(3): 917–940.

陈前恒、林海、吕之望 (2014)。村庄民主能够增加幸福吗?《经济学季刊》, 13 (2) : 723–44.

黄有光 (2013)。人类婚姻有前途吗?评俞炜华的《婚恋与选择》,《经济学家茶座》, 总第59期, 129–132.

Open Access This chapter is licensed under the terms of the Creative Commons Attribution 4.0 International License (http://creativecommons.org/licenses/by/4.0/), which permits use, sharing, adaptation, distribution and reproduction in any medium or format, as long as you give appropriate credit to the original author(s) and the source, provide a link to the Creative Commons license and indicate if changes were made.

The images or other third party material in this chapter are included in the chapter's Creative Commons license, unless indicated otherwise in a credit line to the material. If material is not included in the chapter's Creative Commons license and your intended use is not permitted by statutory regulation or exceeds the permitted use, you will need to obtain permission directly from the copyright holder.

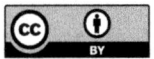

Chapter 11
How Do You Increase Your Happiness?

Abstract Expanding factors already discussed in previous chapters, this chapter identified 12 factors/ways important for increasing happiness: Attitude, balance, confidence, dignity, engagement, family/friends, gratitude, health, ideals, joyful, kindness, love.

Pooling the views of many experts on the useful ways to increase happiness, Buettner et al. (2020, Abstract) conclude that '*Policy strategies* deemed the most effective and feasible are: (1) investing in happiness research, (2) support of vulnerable people and (3) improving the social climate, in particular by promoting voluntary work and supporting non-profits. *Individual strategies* deemed most effective are: (a) investing in social networks, (b) doing meaningful things and (c) caring for one's health.' Public policies for happiness promotion are discussed in Chap. 14 below. Here, we discuss what individuals may do.

While we have mentioned the four F's of happiness (faith, fitness, family, friends) above, these may be increased to 12 factors from A to L, as important factors for and ways one may increase happiness, as discussed below.

First, A is for attitude. An appropriate, positive attitude to life is very important for happiness for oneself as well as for the society. Though happiness is the only thing of intrinsic value (Chap. 5), pursuing only one's own happiness is not the appropriate attitude. This is true not only socially speaking, but also for the individual as well. We have already discussed before that we are born and brought up having happiness in helping others and contributing to the society. It also increases our self-esteem. Confucius said, 'A gentleman is honest and magnanimous; a villain often feels sad'. Being good to the society typically also brings happiness to oneself. This is consistent with modern happiness studies showing that those less purely self-interested, and are willing to help others and providing uncompensated services, are happier (Frey and Stutzer 2002; Bruni and Stanca 2008; Lu et al. 2020; Son and Padilla-Walker 2020).

B is for balance (moderation, the golden mean). This principle is applicable to many areas. Even on the attitude towards time, a balanced view is positive for happiness (Zhang et al. 2013). Even towards the enemies, we should not be excessive; even towards our children, we should not dote on them too much. We should have sufficient exercise, but not too much. Professional sports persons usually do not live long. We should work well, but not too long hours. Excessive working hours are very detrimental to happiness; excessive leisure time is also not good (Haller et al. 2013; de Zeeuw 2018; Lee et al. 2020; Noda 2020). Harmonious (instead of obsessive) 'passion for work may play a salient role in individuals' well-being' (Yukhymenko-Lescroart and Sharma 2019).

Decades ago, I had a colleague who was a workaholic. We share a same secretary who told me that he was working 12 h a day and 7 days a week. This is more than twice my weekly hours of work. True, if we take the total time I am in my office plus the time I work at home over the weekend, it adds up to be more than 50 h. However, some of the office hours are spent on personal affairs like emailing my daughters, my investment agents, etc., not to mention watching beautiful girls on the computer! Haha! Taking off those hours will leave no more than about 40 h. Working in excess of 80 h a week, that colleague of mine not only caused serious family problems at home (I was even called upon to help resolve some), but he eventually died young at 55. The excessive hours did not pay off, even in terms of the narrow result of productivity, not to mention the toll on happiness and his life. (On the desirability of living a balanced life, especially between doing and being, and between relationship and solitude, see Littman-Ovadia 2019. For the importance of modesty, as the balance between arrogance and self-abasement, see Zheng and Wu 2020: 'The more modest you are, the happier you are'.)

C is for confidence. One should have confidence in oneself, and be confident about the future. This is neither being arrogant, nor being blindly optimistic. Rather, it is being cautiously optimistic, recognizing both the subjective (conditions of oneself) and objective factors. Do not have an inferiority complex about oneself. Every person has some advantages and some shortcomings. For example, you may think that I am able to publish many books and papers in top journals, but I also have many aspects much lower than the average. For one thing, I am only 1.6 m in height. After fully grown up, one cannot increase one's height any more. Thus, just take this as given and not to worry about it. I do not aspire to be a basketball star; this is not a problem. As a child, we lived close to the seaside. We went to play in the water since about the age of 3–4. Many of my fellow children of about the same age soon learned how to swim quite well. They could then swim out to the deeper parts of the sea and stay there for an hour or so before coming back. I could not even float. Then another group of younger children joined us. Long after the second or third groups were able to swim to the deeper parts before I managed to float. I never dare to swim to areas deeper than my chest. But again there is no problem as I do not aspire to be an Olympic swimming champion. I started drinking tea and coffee since a young child. However, I could not tell the difference between tea of good and low quality; I could only tell the difference between tea and coffee! Haha! Only until my early 40's, more than three decades since first drinking, that I started to appreciate the difference between high and low qualities, in tea only. Not yet in coffee! At least not much. Also not yet in wines. I find about half of the cheaper types of wines taste good and half not good; and the same proportion for wines 10 times more expensive.

D is for dignity. A person should live with dignity and not doing things bad. Doing bad things may lead to some financial gains in the short run, but losing the more important dignity. Even if others do now know, you know yourself and hence has a lower self-esteem, not to mention the worry of being found out and penalized accordingly. However, the principle of balance, insistance on dignity should not be too extreme. Quite often, stepping back a few steps allows much more scope for both sides. Accepting what is unavoidable saves many troubles. There is no need to quibble on every detail.

E is for engagement. We are a social animal and are born to derive high happiness engaging in interpersonal relationships. Sharing our happiness with family members, friends, relatives, colleagues, etc., we increase, instead of reducing our happiness, while they also typically are also happy sharing it; on the other hand, talking over your sorrows with some good friends usually reduces your unhappiness dramatically, while your friends also feel happy being able to help you reducing your sorrows. Due to our social nature, engaging in socially useful activities usually increases our happiness. According to data from World Values Survey, happiness is highly related to time engaged in interpersonal relationships and voluntary social services (Bruni and Stanca 2008), while the termination of such relationships (divorce or parents' divorce) has very large negative effects on happiness (Helliwell 2003; Dolan et al. 2008).

Engagement is not confined to that on social activities. Just being engaged in doing activities one is interested in may also increases happiness (Lyubomirsky 2008; Lyubomirsky and Layous 2013; Lauzon and Green-Demers 2020).[1] However, many may have spent too much time just watching TV. As this is an easy way to spend time and usually immediate rewards at negligible costs, many may then fail to engage in other activities that are really more rewarding in the long run (Frey et al. 2007). However, Bayraktaroglu et al. (2019) show that watching TV does not reduce happiness the next day, but reduced positive affect increases TV watching the next day.

F is for family and friends. As we have discussed these in the previous chapter, we will skip to G.

G is for gratitude. People in China have a very long tradition of emphasizing the importance of showing gratitude to those who have helped us and repay them when possible. 'A drop of favor should be repaid with a whole spring of water'. The importance of gratitude for happiness is also supported by modern happiness studies (e.g. McCullough et al., 2002; Ruini & Vescovelli 2013; Ahrens & Forbes, 2014; Green et al., 2019; Bohlmeijer et al., 2020); 'feelings of gratitude were positively related to well-being at the within-person level' (Nezlek et al., 2019, Abstract); 'gratitude may not only have a negative influence on depression, but may also counteract the symptoms of depression by enhancing a state of peace of mind' (Liang et al. 2020, Abstract).

We should be grateful not only for those who helped us, but also, if not more so, to those who brought us into being, our parents who typically also have fed and

---

[1] Lauzon and Green-Demers (2020, Abstract) call it 'Savouring ... the capacity to focus on pleasant experiences in order to intensify and prolong the experience of positive affectivity. On the savouring strategies of different age groups, see Marques-Pinto et al. (2020).

educate us, and sacrificed much for us in many other ways. Those who believe in God should also be grateful to God. Those not believing in God should read Ng (2019). In this short book, using five compelling axioms, I prove that God evolved in the wider universe and created our sub-universe about 13.8 billion years ago in the Big Bang (or one identical to it). This explains what Science and Religion have no answer. Science argues for the Big Bang but cannot explain how it came from; religion believes that God created all, but cannot explain how God came about. This little book explains the origins of both our universe and God, its creator. It even answers the question: How came the wider universe? It answers all these questions in ways consistent with what we know now and also logically consistent.

H is for health. We have already discussed this a bit (fitness, one of the 4 F's of happiness). Here, I want to add some more, starting with correcting this mistake: I know the importance of exercising to keep healthy, but I have no time. Instead, for those not lacking time, exercising is not very important; for those not having enough time, exercising is very important.

Compared with no exercising, if you spend half or one hour everyday exercising, you may sleep less by the same amount of time and still wake up fresher the next day, being able to do better quality work and enjoy life better the next day. Thus, exercising actually does not take up time, but earns you time. This is especially so in the long run, as keeping healthy allows you to live a longer life. Studies show that, before an excessive level, each hour of exercise prolongs you live by 2–3 h. The positive effects of exercising on health is clear (Huang and Humphreys 2012; Ruegsegger and Booth 2018; Zhang and Chen 2019). The positive relationship between health and happiness is likely mutual: being healthy increases happiness; being happy is also good for your health (Kim et al. 2013; Trudel-Fitzgerald et al. 2014; Boehm et al. 2017; Lambiase et al. 2015; Martin-Maria et al. 2016; Makki and Mohanty 2019; Steptoe 2019).

Apart from exercising, a healthy lifestyle is also very important for health and happiness, including health food, enough sleep, and a positive attitude (see A for Attitude above) are all relevant. Blanchflower et al. (2013) confirm the general belief that eating more fruits and vegetables are good for health; the optimal amount is no less than seven serves (an apple is one serve) a day (Cf. Mujcic and Oswald 2016). Having enough sunlight is also good for health and happiness (Kaempfer and Mutz 2013).

On healthy food, many years ago, people were very scared of food with high cholesterol. I had a colleague at Monash University who stopped all food with high cholesterol after his hospitalization on some heart problem. A few years later, we heard that he was sent back to hospital for having too few cholesterols. Then, a distinction was made between good and bad cholesterol. However, since a few years ago, even bad cholesterol is OK. Eggs including egg yoke with very high cholesterol are now health food. So is fat meat. In fact, Taubes (2007) argued more than a dozen years ago that cholesterols and fat are not the problem; rather excessive sugar and inadequate fibers are the culprit. This is why sweet potatoes are now on top of the list of heath food.

Around a century ago, at least in Southern China, sweet potatoes are the staple food of the poor; only the rich can afford the more expensive rice. As my mother told us, when some poor people get financially better off, they changed to eating rice. After a few days or weeks, they developed constipation or even haemorrhoids (piles). They then had to change back eating sweet potatoes. Thus they said, 'We are born to eat sweet potatoes [cheap food]!' Of course, it is not the case that some people are born to eat cheap food. Rather, it is the lack of fibers. Even if you can afford it, there is no need to eat and use expensive things; extra money may be donated for altruistic purposes. (On how to do altruism effectively, see MacAskill 2015).

This reminds me about the true story about chicken and lobsters. In the Nineteen Century, lobsters were so plentiful that they were fed only to the poor and prisoners. Prisoners demanded and servants asked for clauses limiting the feeding of lobsters to them at no more than three times a week. The lobster was considered among the least desirable foods, 'a garbage meat fit only for the indigent, indentured, and incarcerated'. (See, e.g. Wallace 2005.) In contrast, chicken was a delicacy affordable only by the rich. Now, with lobsters becoming very scarce and chicken cheap, lobsters become food for the rich people, and chicken as the food for the poor. To some extent, this suggests that if extreme poverty is avoided (no one is starving or very undernourished), some inequality is probably not too serious a matter. Letting the rich pay high prices for items like lobsters, first-class tickets, and luxury skyboxes (for watching sports) helps to some extent to pay for the costs of supply and hence allows others to pay less for other items.

I is for ideal. Every person should have one or more ideals. When a high-school student, my ideal then was to help establish a communist society, believing that it was a more just and happy society. Three events helped me to see the naivety of this belief. First, despite my initial interests in physics, maths and philosophy, I chose to study economics at university, believing that that knowledge would be more relevant in building a new society. However, the study of economics helped me see that capitalism has its rationale, though it may need some government functions to increase equality and deal with environmental disruption. Secondly, the Sino-Soviet dispute over the period about 1958–69 revealed to me further the conceptual and practical problems of communism. Thirdly, the failure of the Great Leap Forward Movement in China over 1958–60 that turned into a great leap downward, and the Cultural Revolution over 1966–76 that bestowed a tremendous amount of hardship on the people, made me realize the impracticability of communism. I thus gave up fighting for communism completely and devote myself to teaching and research.

Not all persons need to have grand ideals which typically turn out impracticable anyway as in my case. It is good to have realistic ideals that are likely realizable. For example, one may wish to be healthy, happy, and successful in career. Some may aspire to be a great entrepreneur or a great scientist. Ideals may be quite high, but should avoid being too unrealistic. If it proves to be unrealizable, one should adjust accordingly. If you cannot be a great entrepreneur, being a successful business person is also good; if you fail to become another Einstein, being a good teacher is also good. As long as you do not cause serious damages to others or the society, and can be happy doing what sustain your life, you should regard yourself as being successful in having largely fulfilling the originally higher ideals.

Having ideals, one will derive much happiness in working towards the achievement of these ideals. Even in my case where I had to give up the original unrealistic ideal, I was very happy while working for it.

In choosing what ideals one should have and work for, three important points should be taken into consideration. First, you should look at your own conditions, your advantages and disadvantages. If you are as short as me, do not aspire to be a basketball champion. Everyone has some comparative advantages. Develop in these directions. Secondly, you must look at the objective situation and find out where you may succeed with your subjective conditions. Thirdly, you must choose something that is beneficial both to yourself and to the society (especially including people around you), usually both financially and happiness wise. Working only for others with no self-benefit is difficult to persist for long, and also not effective. Doing what benefits only yourself but not others will also not last long and achieve big. In the long run, it will usually be counter-productive even to your own interests. Doing something good for both oneself and others will likely promote mutual interaction, complementation, and assistance, and will lead to many more fruitful results.

J is for joyful. Whether a person is usually joyful or not, may to some extent decided by the inborn characters and the experience in one's growing environment and interpersonal relationship. However, one's characters are not completely unchangeable (Boyce et al. 2013). To some extent, we may also try to make ourselves more joyful. One simple way is to avoid going to places that may make you sad, or persons who may make you unhappy. On the other hand, we may do something we enjoy, read something interesting, or watch something amusing. Also, remind oneself to be more joyful and not worry unnecessarily.

K is for kindness. Mencius said, everyone has compassion/kindness, justice, respect/courtesy, wisdom (仁、义、礼、智); these capabilities are in born. At least, there are large inborn components, though not precluding influences of nurture. These capabilities are beneficial to interpersonal cooperation good for our survival.[2] Partly because of the inborn nature and partly because of long-run interaction effects, being kind to others will usually make us happy ourselves. On the beneficial effects of loving-kindness, even just thinking about it, see Gentile et al. (2020). We should be kind not only to our fellow human beings, but also to other animals that may have affective feelings of happiness and pain (the final Chap. 16).

---

[2] On the biological basis of the emotional and moral sentiments, see Konner 2002, Hauser 2006. On the fairness feeling and behaviour of monkeys see Brosnan & de Waal 2003. In humans, Richard Epstein and other scientists in Israel discovered the significant relationships of altruistic behaviour with the Dopamine D4 Receptor gene (Bachner-Melman et al. 2005). The fairness feeling and behaviour also disappear with the electrical interference of the dorsolateral prefrontal cortex (Knoch et al. 2006). Religious or similar beliefs may enhance social relationships, and are beneficial for survival. On the existence of the so-called God gene (DRD4) and the generation of the mystical religious feeling of oneness with the universe, see Persinger (1987), Hamer (2005), Comings (2008), Tiger & McGuire (2010). See also, Johnstone et al. (2017), Ferguson et al. (2018).

L is for love. We have already discussed this in reference to family and marriage above.

References

AHRENS, A. H. & Forbes, C. N. (2014). Gratitude. In TUGADE, M. M., SHIOTA, M. N., KIRBY, L. D. (Eds.), *Handbook of positive emotions*, pp. 342–361, New York: Guilford Press.

BACHNER-MELMAN, R., GRITSENKO, I., NEMANOV, L., ZOHAR, A. H., DINA, C. & EBSTEIN, R. P. (2005). Dopaminergic polymorphisms associated with self-report measures of human altruism: A fresh phenotype for the dopamine D4 receptor. *Molecular Psychiatry*, 10: 333-5.

BAYRAKTAROGLU, D., GUNAYDIN, G., SELCUK, E. et al. (2019). A Daily Diary Investigation of the Link Between Television Watching and Positive Affect. *Journal of Happiness Studies, 20*(4), 1089–1101. https://doi.org/10.1007/s10902-018-9989-8.

BLANCHFLOWER, D. G., OSWALD, A. J. & STEWART-BROWN, S. (2013). Is psychological well-being linked to the consumption of fruit and vegetables? *Social Indicators Research, 114*(3), 785–801.

BOEHM, Julia K., KIM, Eric S. & KUBZANSKY, Laura, D. (2017). *Positive psychological wellbeing*. Routledge.

BOHLMEIJER, E. T., KRAISS, J. T., WATKINS, P. et al. (2020). Promoting Gratitude as a Resource for Sustainable Mental Health: Results of a 3-Armed Randomized Controlled Trial up to 6 Months Follow-up. *Journal of Happiness Studies*. https://doi.org/10.1007/s10902-020-00261-5.

BOYCE, C. J., WOOD, A. M. & POWDTHAVEE, N. (2013). Is personality fixed? Personality changes as much as "variable" economic factors and more strongly predicts changes to life satisfaction. *Social Indicators Research, 111*(1), 287–305.

BROSNAN, Sarah F. & DE WAAL, Frans B. M. (2003). Monkeys reject unequal pay, *Nature*, 425: 297-299. Doi: 10.1038/nature01963

BRUNI, L. & STANCA, L. (2008). Watching alone relational goods, television and happiness. *Journal of Economic Behavior & Organization, 65*, 506–528.

BUETTNER, D., NELSON, T. & VEENHOVEN, R. (2020). Ways to greater happiness: A Delphi study. *Journal of Happiness Studies*. https://doi.org/10.1007/s10902-019-00199-3.

COMINGS, David E. (2008). *Did Man Creat God?* Duarte, CA: Hope

DE ZEEUW, N. (2018). The effect of working hours on subjective well-being. Corpus ID: 149479435. Retrieved from: https://www.semanticscholar.org/paper/The-Effect-of-Working-Hours-on-Subjective-Zeeuw/71eefdd3b1c67da0fb99dad75dd748af2f8ae0b0.

DOLAN, P., PEASGOOD, T. & WHITE, M. (2008). Do you really know what makes us happy? A review of the economic literature on the factors associated with subjective well-being. *Journal of Economic Psychology, 29*, 94–122.

EPSTEIN, Richard A. (2018). The Dangerous allure of libertarian paternalism. *Review of Behavioral Economics, 5*(3-4), 389-416.

FERGUSON, Michael A., et al. Reward, salience, and attentional networks are activated by religious experience in devout Mormons. *Social neuroscience*, 2018, 13(1), 104-116.

FREY, Bruno S. & STUTZER, Alois (2002). What can economists learn from happiness research? *Journal of Economic Literature*, 40: 402-35.

FREY, Bruno S., BENESCH, C. & STUTZER, A. (2007). Does watching TV make us happy? *Journal of Economic psychology, 28*(3), 283–313.

JOHNSTONE, Brick, et al. (2017). Selflessness as a universal neuropsychological foundation of spiritual transcendence: validation with Christian, Hindu, and Muslim traditions. *Mental Health, Religion & Culture, 20*(2), 175–187.

GENTILE, D. A., SWEET, D. M. & HE, L. (2020). Caring for Others Cares for the Self: An Experimental Tes. t of Brief Downward Social Comparison, Loving-Kindness, and Interconnectedness Contemplations. *Journal of Happiness Studies, 21*, 765–778. https://doi.org/10.1007/s10 902-019-00100-2.

GREEN, Z.A., NOOR, U. & AHMED, F. (2019). The body–mind–spirit dimensions of wellness mediate dispositional gratitude and life satisfaction. *Journal of Happiness Studies.* https://doi.org/10.1007/s10902-019-00215-6.

HALLER, Max, HADLER, Markus & KAUP, Gerd (2013). Leisure time in modern societies: A new source of boredom and stress? *Social Indicators Research,* 111(2): 403-434.

HAMER, D. C. (2005). *The God Gene.* New York: Anchor Books.

HAUSER, Marc D. (2006). *Moral Minds: How Nature Designed Our Universal Sense of Right and Wrong.* New York: Harper Collins.

HELLIWELL, JOHN F. (2003). How's life? Combining individual and national variables to explain subjective well-being. *Economic Modelling, 20*(2), 331–360.

HUANG, Haifang & HUMPHREYS, Brad R. (2012). Sports participation and happiness: Evidence from US microdata. *Journal of Economic Psychology,* 33(4): 776-93.

KAEMPFER, Sylvia & MUTZ, Michael (2013). On the sunny side of life: Sunshine effects on life satisfaction. *Social Indicators Research,* 110(2): 579–95.

KIM ES, SUN JK, PARK N, PETERSON C. (2013). Purpose in life and reduced incidence of stroke in olderadults: 'The Health and Retirement Study. *Journal of Psychosomatic Research, 74*, 427–432.

KNOCH, Daria, et al. (2006). Diminishing reciprocal fairness by disrupting the right prefrontal cortex. *Science,* 314(5800): 829-32. DOI:10.1126/science.1129156.

KONNER, Melvin (2002). *The Tangled Wing: Biological Constraints on the Human Spirit.* New York: Henry Holt.

LAMBIASE MJ, KUBZANSKY LD, THURSTON RC. (2015). Positive psychological health and stroke risk: Thebenefits of emotional vitality. *Health Psychology, 34*, 1043–1046.

LAUZON, A. & GREEN-DEMERS, I. (2020). More of a Good Thing is Even Better: Towards a New Conceptualization of the Nature of Savouring Experiences. *Journal of Happiness Studies, 21*(4), 1225–1249. https://doi.org/10.1007/s10902-019-00125-7.

LEE, K. J., CHO, S., KIM, E. K., et al. (2020). Do More Leisure Time and Leisure Repertoire Make Us Happier? An Investigation of the Curvilinear Relationships. *Journal of Happiness Studies, 21*(5), 1727–1747. https://doi.org/10.1007/s10902-019-00153-3.

LIANG, H., CHEN, C., LI, F., WU, S., WANG, L., ZHENG, X. & ZENG, B. (2020). Mediating effects of peace of mind and rumination on the relationship between gratitude and depression among Chinese university students. *Current Psychology, 39*, 1430–1437. https://doi.org/10.1007/s12144-018-9847-1.

LITTMAN-OVADIA, H. (2019). Doing–being and relationship–solitude: A proposed model for a balanced life. *Journal of Happiness Studies, 20*(6), 1953–1971. https://doi.org/10.1007/s10902-018-0018-8.

LU, C., JIANG, Y., ZHAO, X. et al. (2020). Will helping others also benefit you? Chinese adolescents' altruistic personality traits and life satisfaction. *Journal of Happiness Studies, 21*(4), 1407–1425. https://doi.org/10.1007/s10902-019-00134-6.

LYUBOMIRSKY, Sonja & LAYOUS, Kristin. (2013). How do simple positive activities increase well-being? *Psychological Science, 22*, 57–62.

LYUBOMIRSKY, Sonja. (2008). *The How of Happiness: A Scientific Approach to Getting the Life You Want.* Penguin.

MACASKILL, William. (2015). *Doing Good Better: How Effective Altruism Can Help You Make a Difference.* Guardian.

MAKKI, N. & MOHANTY, M. S. (2019). Mental health and happiness: Evidence from the US data. *The American Economist,* 0569434518822266.

References

MARQUES-PINTO, A., OLIVEIRA, S., SANTOS, A. et al. (2020). Does our age affect the way we live? A study on savoring strategies across the life span. *Journal of Happiness Studies, 21*, 1509–1528. https://doi.org/10.1007/s10902-019-00136-4.

MARTIN-MARIA, N., CABALLERO, F., OLAYA, B., et al. (2016). Positive affect is inversely associated with mortality in individuals without depression. *Frontiers in Psychology, 7*, 1040. https://doi.org/10.3389/fpsyg.2016.01040.

MCCULLOUGH, M. E., EMMONS, R. A. & TSANG, J. (2002). The grateful disposition: A conceptual and empirical topography. *Journal of Personality and Social Psychology, 82*(1), 112–127. https://doi.org/10.1037/0022-3514.82.1.112.d.

MUJCIC, Redzo, and OSWALD, Andrew J. (2016). Evolution of well-being and happiness after increases in consumption of fruit and vegetables. *American journal of public health* 106(8): 1504-1510.

NEZLEK, J.B., KREJTZ, I., RUSANOWSKA, M. et al. (2019). Within-person relationships among daily gratitude, well-being, stress, and positive experiences. *Journal of Happiness Studies, 20*(3), 883–898. https://doi.org/10.1007/s10902-018-9979-x.

NG, Yew-Kwang (2019). *Evolved-God Creationism: A View of How God Evolved in the Wider Universe*, Cambridge Scholars.

NODA, H. (2020). Work-Life Balance and Life Satisfaction in OECD Countries: A Cross-Sectional Analysis. *Journal of Happiness Studies, 21*, 1325–1348. https://doi.org/10.1007/s10902-019-00131-9.

PERSINGER, M. (1987). Neurobiological Bases of God Beliefs. New York: Praeger.

RUEGSEGGER, G. N. & BOOTH, F. W. (2018). Health benefits of exercise. *Cold Spring Harbor perspectives in medicine, 8*(7), a029694.

RUINI, Chiara & VESCOVELLI, Francesca. (2013). The role of gratitude in breast cancer: Its relationships with post-traumatic growth, psychological well-being and distress. *Journal of Happiness Studies, 14*(1), 263–274.

SON, D. & PADILLA-WALKER, L.M. (2020). Happy helpers: A multidimensional and mixed-method approach to prosocial behavior and its effects on friendship quality, mental health, and well-being during adolescence. Journal of Happiness Studies 21(5): 1705–1723, 1725. https://doi.org/10.1007/s10902-019-00154-2.

STEPTOE, Andrew (2019). Happiness and health, *Annual Review of Public Health*.

TAUBES, Gary. (2007). *Good Calories*. Knopf.

TIGER, Lionel & MCGUIRE, Michael (2010). *God's Brain*. Amherst: Prometheus.

TRUDEL-FITZGERALD, C., BOEHM, J. K., KIVIMAKI, M., KUBZANSKY, L. D. (2014). Taking the tension out of hypertension: A prospective study of psychological well-being and hypertension. *Journal of Hypertension, 32*, 1222–1228.

WALLACE, David F. (2005). *Consider the Lobster and Other Essays*, Little, Brown & Co.

YUKHYMENKO-LESCROART, M. A. & SHARMA, G. (2019). The relationship between faculty members' passion for work and well-being. *Journal of Happiness Studies, 20*(3), 863–881.

ZHANG, Z. & CHEN, W. A. (2019). Systematic review of the relationship between physical activity and happiness. *Journal of Happiness Studies, 20*(4), 1305–1322. https://doi.org/10.1007/s10902-018-9976-0.

ZHANG, Jia Wei, HOWELL, Ryan T. & STOLARSKI, Maciej (2013). Comparing three methods to measure a balanced time perspective: The relationship between a balanced time perspective and subjective well-being. *Journal of Happiness Studies, 14*(1): 169-84.

ZHENG, C. & WU, Y. (2020). The more modest you are, the happier you are: The mediating roles of emotional intelligence and self-esteem. *Journal of Happiness Studies, 21*(5), 1603–1615. https://doi.org/10.1007/s10902-019-00144-4.

Open Access This chapter is licensed under the terms of the Creative Commons Attribution 4.0 International License (http://creativecommons.org/licenses/by/4.0/), which permits use, sharing, adaptation, distribution and reproduction in any medium or format, as long as you give appropriate credit to the original author(s) and the source, provide a link to the Creative Commons license and indicate if changes were made.

The images or other third party material in this chapter are included in the chapter's Creative Commons license, unless indicated otherwise in a credit line to the material. If material is not included in the chapter's Creative Commons license and your intended use is not permitted by statutory regulation or exceeds the permitted use, you will need to obtain permission directly from the copyright holder.

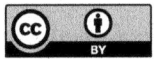

Chapter 12
Stimulating Our Brains and Transforming Our Selves

Abstract The stimulation of the pleasure centres in our brain by electricity or other means induces intense pleasures. Despite its discovery for nearly seven decades, this method has not been widely used and discussed. Relatively small investment in perfecting this technique would give us a device for achieving easy and 'supra-maximal' pleasure that would obliviate pain, depression, and replace harmful drugs. With adequate safeguards, we could also use genetic engineering to transform ourselves and make us much more capable of happiness, surpassing the 'supra-maximal' pleasure of brain stimulation.

Apart from the normal ways to increase our happiness discussed in the previous chapters, there are other ways opened up by science and technology. Moreover, these new ways may increase our happiness by many times more than the traditional methods. First, for the traditional methods, including some technological advances in the past like the invention of television, their contributions to happiness are subject to the serious limitation of adaptation, losing their novelty and high marginal utilities very quickly. While the adaptation effect will no doubt also dilute the welfare significance of such innovations as web-surfing, there are at least two areas of expected future advance that will not be significantly subject to the satiation (applying at the moment of consumption) and adaptation (applying in the longer run) effects. Instead, they are likely capable of increasing our happiness by x times rather than x%, where x is a large number.

12.1 Stimulating the Pleasure Centers in Our Brains

First, there is the stimulation of the pleasure centres in our brain. It has been known for more than six decades that deep brain stimulation (DBS) with electricity or other means[1] can relieve acute pain, induce intense pleasure, and promote a

---
[1] Apart from using electricity, there are other ways, including magnetic and ultrasound, of direct stimulation of the brain's pleasure centers; see e.g. Reti (2015), Frank (2018), Harmsen et al. (2018), Moisset et al. (2020).

sense of well-being without the undesirable health effects of drug addiction.[2] There have been research experiments and medical therapies in using DBS, especially in treating Parkinson's disease (e.g. Cai et al. 2020), depression (e.g. Coenen et al. 2018; Kisely et al. 2018; Liu et al. 2020), and post-traumatic stress disorder (e.g. Koek et al. 2019). However, the enormous potential benefits of DBS have neither been adequately explored nor widely discussed. Much increased research effort and eventual widespread use of DBS are called for.

Positive reward associated with DBS leading to voluntary self-stimulation was discovered by Olds and Milner (1954) when they observed that a rat returned to the place where it received direct electrical stimulation of certain parts of its brain. Further research established sites that induce pleasure (medial forebrain bundle, septal, limbic and hypothalamic areas), pain, and ambiguous or mixed feelings. Stimulation of the pleasurable sites clearly produces positive reward as suggested by experiments in which rats were willing to cross a painful shock grid in order to obtain the stimulation, and as confirmed by human subjects. Moreover, the pleasure induced is so intense that rats prefer DBS to food and sex, and if not stopped by experimenters, will continuously seek stimulation until exhaustion. In humans, *'patients who were having emotional or physical pain experienced such intense pleasure with stimulation that the pain was obliterated'* (Heath et al. 1968, p. 188). Scholars describe the feeling from brain stimulation as 'super–pleasure or 'supramaximal' (Dror 2016.)

Apart from relieving pain and inducing pleasure, DBS may also be used as a 'primer' in improving well-being. For example, Heath (1964, p. 236) reported, '*strong pleasure* [from brain stimulation] *was associated with sexual feelings, and in most instances the patient experienced spontaneous orgasm … This patient, now married to her third husband, had never experienced orgasm before she received … stimulation to the brain, but since then has consistently achieved climax during sexual relations.*' Once the right neurons have been excited, they become excitable more easily. The right neural pathways have been established.

Among the important social problems of our time are drug addiction, crimes and (mental) depression. These social problems, and possibly others, seem to be largely solvable with the widespread use of DBS. In comparison to DBS, the use of addictive drugs like heroin is a very inefficient and dangerous method of achieving a 'high'. If one has easy access to intensely pleasurable sensations by just turning on the electricity, there seems little reason left to try dangerous alternatives like heroin. Just as intractable pain may be relieved by DBS, mental depression should also be largely removable by positive DBS. Since most depressions are caused by failure to achieve happiness one way or other, the availability of happy sensations by DBS should provide a definite relief. Among others, the amelioration of stress (Patterson et al. 1994), reduction of stress ulcers (Yadin and Thomas 1996), improved performance in maze (Jiang et al. 1997), and the treatment of alcoholics (Krupitskii et al. 1993) have been reported.

---

[2] There are also other benefits such as improving sleep quality (Dafsari et al. 2020) and vision restoration (Gall et al. 2013).

Though DBS is not physically addictive, it might be psychologically addictive. However, in contrast to heroin addiction, DBS addiction is not dangerous to health. From the quite large amount of evidence we have, the proper use (Kavirajan et al. 2014; Patterson and Kesner 1981; Zhang et al. 2020) of DBS over a sustained period for a long time (e.g. a few hours daily over a number of years) has proved to be efficacious and safe.[3] Thus DBS addiction is only a problem if it leads to the serious disregard of other duties such as to threaten the welfare of (mainly) other people (especially the future generations). While the pleasures induced by DBS can be intense, I doubt that psychological addiction of such a magnitude would occur. Rats choose to use DBS until exhaustion but humans only for "up to half an hour daily" (Sem-Jacobsen, reported in Delgado 1976, p. 484). Relative to other pleasures and objectives, the pleasure of DBS does not seem to be compelling for humans (Bishop et al. 1964; Valenstein 1973, p. 28). If one believes in creation, perhaps God made us this way so that we could eventually provide happiness not only for ourselves but also for animals. In the unlikely event of serious addiction, the problem could be solved by using legal and/or technical devices restricting the unlimited use of DBS. For example, the electricity that could be used for brain stimulation is supplied over certain limited hours only.

While DBS addiction is unlikely to be so serious as to threaten the survival of a civilized society, it may be feared that it would significantly reduce mutual human relationships. If one could obtain pleasure by simply turning on the electricity, there might be little motivation left for the cultivation of personal relationships. This is unlikely to happen. Even if one could obtain a variety of pleasurable sensations by DBS, there would still be the innate need for companionship left. Secondly, the pleasure from DBS to humans does not seem to be as fulfilling as, say, a full sexual relationship with its simultaneous stimulation of a number of areas and close personal contact, nor as rewarding as spiritual fulfilment of the highest order. Thirdly, the provision of pleasure which might otherwise be unavailable in sufficient amount may in fact create many happy and easy-to-go-with individuals. This may remove many personal conflicts and promote better mutual relationships. Fourthly, even if personal relationships were reduced, the benefits of DBS would still likely to much more than compensate for the loss. For example, the introduction of television probably has significantly reduced conversation. But that does not necessarily make it a bad thing. Its benefits have to be taken into account as well.

In this connection, the long-lasting nature of pleasure from DBS definitely gives it a big advantage. Things like television usually appear to have enormous potential benefits around the time of their initial introduction. After prolonged usage, some of their disadvantages are discovered though some other beneficial usages may also be found. More importantly, the novelty value has disappeared. For example, while watching television is very enjoyable for those just getting access to it, it may become a second best option after its novelty value has disappeared. The benefits of television

---

[3] For some side effects of DBS, see Schüpbach, et al. (2006), Christen et al. (2012) and Gallagher (2021). However, 'the results of DBS treatment are mostly positive' (Gallagher 2021, p.32); Cf. Voigt (2021) on the positive aspects of DBS.

probably still outweigh its costs by a very wide margin, but not by as much as it would be if the novelty value could be maintained. With DBS, the situation would be different. Since DBS is the ***direct*** stimulation of the brain, the pleasure during stimulation does not depend on any novelty value. Moreover, the intensity of pleasure from DBS does not diminish with prolonged stimulation (either continuously or daily over a number of years). Our hypothalamus where pleasure is produced continue to respond normally to stimulation many thousand times unabated. Thus, there is no diminishing marginal utility in DBS.

Common methods of enjoyment through the stimulation of our senses (through the peripheral nervous systems) like eating delicious food and having sex is, after some point, subject to fast diminishing marginal returns. This is so because we are programmed through natural selection to protect us from over-eating, etc. On the other hand, activities that yields no significant diminishing marginal returns such as reading typically produces low levels of reward at each moment. This is so since these activities had not been very essential over our long evolutionary history in increasing our selection fitness. True, humans are capable of higher levels of happiness including spiritual fulfillment. If it is not the only species on Earth that is capable of spiritual feelings, it is certainly the only one where such feelings could be so strong or intense. Nevertheless, even here adaptation and diminishing marginal utility apply quickly. Thus, even the winning of a Nobel prize is said to yield a high for only about two weeks. Thus, our ordinary biological capacity for happiness is rather limited. However, in our eons of evolution, our brain was not stimulated intracranially (bypassing the peripheral nervous systems) and hence there has been no need to program diminishing marginal returns directly within the pleasure centres in our brain. Thus, brain stimulation promises high happiness due to the absence of diminishing marginal utility. Hence, intense pleasure over long duration is possible, and with no apparent harm. For example, a monkey receiving stimulation presses the button three times every second, 16 h a day, several days a week, over many years. Researchers have to arrange it such as to prevent death from starvation or lack of water, not from stimulation. I do not mind being that monkey! Thus the enormous increase in happiness brought about by DBS could be expected to be maintained largely unabated, and in fact could be greatly increased through better techniques of stimulation (Cf. Sathi and Hosain 2020).

DBS may be regarded as unnatural in the sense that it does not occur in the course of our natural biological evolution. But most civilized products, institutions, medical treatments, etc., are unnatural in this sense. This does not make them bad. To improve our welfare, we have invented many "unnatural" things. DBS is a recent invention that if properly made use of widely, possesses welfare significance surpassing all previous inventions put together.

Many people from the West may find, upon first contact, the culture, tradition, and ways of enjoying life in the East and in some primitive tribes degrading. The same is true for people from the East on some Western ways of life. But we have learned from liberalism to be more tolerant towards different cultures and ways of life as long as they are not harmful. Many liberals would go further in tolerating individual freedom of action even for those actions which are harmful to the actors themselves.

DBS is about the least harmful way of inducing intense pleasure and should never be regarded as degrading by anyone who has the slightest adherence to liberalism. (See also Pugh 2020 on the ethical issues of some possible personality changes, existence of which is still being debated.)

Will God approve DBS? If one does not believe in God, the question does not arise (but then he/she should read Ng 2019). If one believes in God, then the answer seems to be affirmative. For example, the ten commandments do not include: Thou shall not engage in DBS! Nor do they include: Thou shall not enjoy yourself. Moreover, if God does not want us to use DBS, why did He create us in a way that DBS can induce intense positive rewards?

If higher funding for research could result in such spectacularly welfare-improving discoveries and inventions as DBS, the present writer would be prepared to halve his post-tax income to help pay for them.

For the 500 million or more of people just in China who have attained the level of reasonable comfort, a further increase of even a hundred thousand (Chinese) dollars each will not increase happiness appreciably at the social level in the long run. However, if these half a billion people contribute just ten dollars each, we will have 5 billion dollars. Alternatively, this sum of money may be allocated by the Chinese government. This amount is less than one in 4 thousands or 0.025% of the foreign exchange reserve of China, and also less than one in twenty thousand or 0.005% of the annual GDP in China. This relatively small sum of money would be enough to fund research to develop a machine or instrument that we may use to stimulate our brain for pleasure safely. The increase in happiness will be many times that of increasing the GDP by ten times. Spreading the result to the rest of the world, China would contribute more than its four ancient innovations combined!

After mass production, each machine will likely not cost more than that of a TV set. If needed, I would be willing to pay millions of dollars to get one. My consumer surplus would likely be many thousand times its price.

After learning of my views on this, a commentator in China emailed me, 'When it comes to experiments on humans, would you be willing to volunteer? Or rather, you would wait until China used its prisoners for experiments to produce the fruit that you Western advisors would enjoy?' I replied to her immediately that I would be glad to volunteer to be the first human guinea pig. I do not see this as being altruistic. Rather, I cannot wait to be that monkey.

12.2 Genetic Engineering and Our Own Transformation

Another expected advance that will lead to dramatic leaps in happiness may be expected in genetic engineering. It is true that here we have to be even more careful than in brain stimulation to avoid being counter-productive. Nevertheless, with care and sufficient safeguards, genetic engineering promises great leaps because it may transform our capacity for enjoyment itself. Short of the extremes like brain stimulation and starvation, the happiness level of a person depends more on the subjective factors than the objective circumstances. The subjective factors are shaped by our upbringings, education, social contacts, and a host of other factors. However, these factors affect mainly the waves of happiness around a set point. The level of this set point for each person is largely genetic (Lykken and Tellegen 1996; Lykken 1999). This does not mean that we cannot affect our happiness levels at all. Even Lykken (1999) who has established the high degree of association of happiness and a host of other things with genetic factors through the study of identical twins (including those reared apart), believes that we can learn to become happier by affecting the waves of happiness. Nevertheless, the dominance of the genetic factors in determining the set points remains. Even with DBS, the degree of the intense pleasure is also set. This suggests that a way to increase happiness by a quantum leap more important than brain stimulation is through genetic engineering. Of course, a very high degree of care has to be taken for such an endeavour. Is it too risky nevertheless? While there are some risks, they could be reduced by sufficient safeguards. Moreover, the risks involved are far less than those created by our current path of high growth without sufficient environmental protection. The returns of this high growth are just some chance (if problems like climate change turn out to be of no significance) of higher output that contributes virtually nothing to happiness. The risks are high chance of environmental disasters including human extinction. In contrast, genetic engineering promises a very high chance of huge quantum leaps in our happiness, at negligible and avoidable risks. Why do many people still feel comfortable with the former and not with the latter? I do not advocate using drastic forms of genetic engineering to transform ourselves right now or even in the near future. However, research on this and its eventual gradual usage with sufficient safeguards should not be precluded.[4]

To put it emphatically, it may be said that mankind is facing the greatest cross-road in its entire history: We may choose to ignore the threat of global warming and choose business as usual and go to Hell (extinction), or we may adequately solve the problem of environmental disruption and ensure our road to Heaven (survival and quantum leaps in the welfare of our offspring). The human species had faced the threat of extinction before. Yet the current cross-road is more remarkable than previous ones for two reasons. First, the current threat is man-made and could be undone by us. Second, if we could avoid the current threat, we will have very good chance of going to Heaven (quantum leaps in welfare). The difference has never been greater!

References

AGGARWAL, S. & CHUGH, N. (2020). Ethical implications of closed loop brain device: 10-year review. *Minds & Machines, 30*, 145–170.

---

[4] Some brain implants and brain-computer interface have achieved clinical successes; see, e.g. Aggarwal and Chugh (2020) on these devices and the related ethical issues.

References

BISHOP, M. P., ELDER, S. T. & HAETH, R. G. (1964). Attempted control of operant behavior in man with intracranial self-stimulation. In HEATH, H. & ROW, (Hoeber)(1964), *The Role of Pleasure in Behavior Robert*, 55–81, New York.

CAI, Y., REDDY, R. D., VARSHNEY, V. et al. (2020). Spinal cord stimulation in Parkinson's disease: A review of the preclinical and clinical data and future prospects. *Bioelectron Med, 6*, 5. https://doi.org/10.1186/s42234-020-00041-9

CHRISTEN, M., BITTLINGER, M., WALTER, H., BRUGGER, P. & MÜLLER, S. (2012). Dealing with side effects of deep brain stimulation: Lessons learned from stimulating the STN. *AJOB Neuroscience, 3*(1), 37–43.

COENEN, V. A., SAJONZ, B. E., REISERT, M., BOSTRÖM, J. P., BEWERNICK, B., URBACH, H., JENKNER, C., REINACHER, P. C., SCHLAEPFER, T. E. & MÄDLER, B. (2018). Tractography-assisted deep brain stimulation of the superolateral branch of the medial forebrain bundle (slMFB DBS) in major depression. *NeuroImage : Clinical, 20*, 580–593. https://doi.org/10.1016/j.nicl.2018.08.020

DAFSARI, H. S., RAY-CHAUDHURI, K., ASHKAN, K. et al. (2020). Beneficial effect of 24-month bilateral subthalamic stimulation on quality of sleep in Parkinson's disease. *Journal of Neurology, 267*, 1830–1841. https://doi.org/10.1007/s00415-020-09743-1

DELGADO, J. M. R. (1976). New orientation in brain stimulation in man. *Brain-stimulation reward*.

DROR, OTNIEL E. (2016). Cold War "super-pleasure": Insatiability, self-stimulation, and the postwar brain. *Osiris, 31*(1), 227–249.

FRANK, Lone (2018). *The Pleasure Shock: The Rise of Deep Brain Stimulation and Its Forgotten Inventor*, New York: Dutton. Also:https://www.theatlantic.com/health/archive/2018/03/pleasure-shock-deep-brain-stimulation-happiness/556043/

GALLAGHER, Shaun (2021). Deep brain stimulation, self and relational autonomy. *Neuroethics, 14*(1), 31-43. doi:http://dx.doi.org/10.1007/s12152-018-9355-x

GALL, C., ANTAL, A. & SABEL, B.A. (2013). Non-invasive electrical brain stimulation induces vision restoration in patients with visual pathway damage. *Graefes Archive for Clinical and Experimental Ophthalmology, 251*, 1041–1043. https://doi.org/10.1007/s00417-012-2084-7

HARMSEN, I. E., ROWLAND, N. C., WENNBERG, R. A. & LOZANO, A. M. (2018). Characterizing the effects of deep brain stimulation with magnetoencephalography: A review. *Brain Stimulation., 11*(3), 481–491.

HEATH, R. G. (Ed.). (1964). *The Role of Pleasure in Behavior*. Harper and Row.

HEATH, Robert G., JOHN, Stanley B. & FONTANA, Charles J (1968). The pleasure response: Studies by stereotaxic technics in patients. In Kline, N. and Laska, E. (Eds.), *Computers and Electronic Devices*, Grune & Stratton, New York.

JIANG, F., RACINE R. & TURNBULL. J. (1997). Electrical stimulation of the septal region of aged rats improves performance in an open-field maze. *Physiology & Behavior, 62*(6), 1279–1282.

KAVIRAJAN, H.C., LUECK, K. & CHUANG, K. (2014). Alternating current cranial electrotherapy stimulation (CES) for depression. The Cochrane database of systematic reviews, 7, CD010521. DOI:https://doi.org/10.1002/14651858.CD010521.pub2

KISELY, S.R., LI, A., WARREN, N. & SISKIND, D.J. (2018). A systematic review and meta-analysis of deep brain stimulation for depression. *Depression and Anxiety, 35*, 468–480. https://doi.org/10.1002/da.22746

KOEK, R.J., ROACH, J., ATHANASIOU, N., WOUT-FRANK, M.V. & PHILIP, N.S. (2019). Neuromodulatory treatments for post-traumatic stress disorder (PTSD). *Progress in Neuro-Psychopharmacology and Biological Psychiatry, 92*, 148–160. https://doi.org/10.1016/j.pnpbp.2019.01.004

KRUPITSKII, E. M., BURAKOV, A. M., KARANDASHOVA, G. F., LEBEDEV, V. B., et al. (1993). A method of treating affective disorders in alcoholics. *Journal of Russian & East European Psychiatry, 26*(3), 26–37.

LIU, C., YANG, M., ZHANG, G., WANG, X., LI, B., LI, M., WOELFER, M., WALTER, M. & WANG, L. (2020). Neural networks and the anti-inflammatory effect of transcutaneous auricular vagus nerve stimulation in depression. Journal of Neuroinflammation, 17. DOI:https://doi.org/10.1186/s12974-020-01732-5

LYKKEN, David (1999). *Happiness: What studies on twins show us about nature, nurture, and the happiness set-point.* Golden Books.

LYKKEN, David & TELLEGEN, Auke. (1996). Happiness is a stochastic phenomenon. *Psychological Science, 7*(3), 186–189.

MOISSET, X., LANTERI-MINET, M. & FONTAINE, D. (2020). Neurostimulation methods in the treatment of chronic pain. *Journal of Neural Transmission, 127,* 673–686. https://doi.org/10.1007/s00702-019-02092-y

NG, Yew-Kwang (2019). *Evolved-God Creationism: A View of How God Evolved in the Wider Universe,* Cambridge Scholars.

OLDS, James & MILNER, Peter. (1954). Positive reinforcement produced by electrical stimulation of septal area and other regions of the rat brain. *Journal of Comparative Physiological Psychology, 47,* 419–427.

PATTERSON, M. M. & KESNER, R. P. (1981). *Electrical Stimulation Research Techniques.* Academic Press.

PATTERSON, M., KRUPITSKY, E., FLOOD, N., and BAKER, D. (1994). Amelioration of stress in chemical dependency detoxification by transcranial electrostimulation. *Stress Medicine, 10*(2), 115–126.

PUGH, Jonathan. (2020). Clarifying the normative significance of 'personality changes' following deep brain stimulation. *Science and Engineering Ethics, 26,* 1655–1680. https://doi.org/10.1007/s11948-020-00207-3

RETI, I. ed. (2015). *Brain Stimulation: Methodologies and Interventions,* John Wiley & Sons.

SATHI, K.A. & HOSAIN, M.K. (2020). Modeling and simulation of deep brain stimulation electrodes with various active contacts. *Res. Biomed. Eng., 36,* 147–161. https://doi.org/10.1007/s42600-020-0000-0

SCHÜPBACH, M., M. GARGIULO, M.L. WELTER, C. MALLET, C. BÉHAR, AND J.L. HOUETO (2006). Neurosurgery in Parkinson disease: A distressed mind in a repaired body? Neurology, 66: 1811–1816. https://doi.org/10.1212/01.wnl.0000234880.51322.16.

VALENSTEIN, A. F. (1973). On attachment to painful feelings and the negative therapeutic reaction. *The Psychoanalytic Study of the Child, 28*(1), 365–392.

VOIGT, Julia S. (2021). Bodily Felt Freedom: an Ethical Perspective on Positive Aspects of Deep Brain Stimulation, Neuroethics, 14:45–57. https://doi.org/10.1007/s12152-018-9380-9

YADIN, Elna, THOMAS, Earl. (1996). Stimulation of the lateral septum attenuates immobilization-induced stress ulcers. *Physiology & Behavior, 59*(4–5), 883–886.

ZHANG, X., QING, M., RAO, Y. & GUO, Y. (2020). Adjunctive vagus nerve stimulation for treatment-resistant depression: A quantitative analysis. Psychiatric Quarterly, 1–11. DOI:https://doi.org/10.1007/s11126-020-09726-5.

Open Access This chapter is licensed under the terms of the Creative Commons Attribution 4.0 International License (http://creativecommons.org/licenses/by/4.0/), which permits use, sharing, adaptation, distribution and reproduction in any medium or format, as long as you give appropriate credit to the original author(s) and the source, provide a link to the Creative Commons license and indicate if changes were made.

The images or other third party material in this chapter are included in the chapter's Creative Commons license, unless indicated otherwise in a credit line to the material. If material is not included in the chapter's Creative Commons license and your intended use is not permitted by statutory regulation or exceeds the permitted use, you will need to obtain permission directly from the copyright holder.

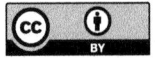

Chapter 13
The East-Asian Happiness Gap: Causes and Implications

Abstract Despite spectacular economic growth, most East Asian countries (especially those with the Confucian cultures) score relatively low in happiness surveys. This chapter discusses the reasons for this East-Asian happiness gap, including environmental disruption, excessive competitiveness, repressive education, excessive conformity, negative attitudes towards enjoyment, and the emphasis on outward appearance. Implications on the desired direction of future growth especially regarding the relative importance of public spending on the environment and research and the non-material aspects of life are also briefly touched on.

13.1 The East-Asian Happiness Gap

The East-Asian countries/regions referred to here include Mainland China, Hong Kong, Taiwan, Korea, Japan, and Singapore. To some extent, it probably also applies to Malaysia and Vietnam, but not much to the Philippines, Thailand, and Indonesia which have rather different cultures.

While East Asia (with the major exception of Japan in the last three decades) has done extremely well economically, it has not done well at all in terms of the ultimate objective of life—happiness. In fact, an older international comparison (Cummins 1998) puts East Asians (China, Japan and Korea) as the very lowest group of countries, after the top group of Northern Europeans, followed by the English-speaking countries, Latin Americans, Southeast Asians, the Middle East, middle Europeans, South-Eastern Europeans, South Asia, Africa, and South-Western Europeans. Singapore had a per-capita income 64 times that of India (and more than 16 times even after PPP adjustment), but had the same happiness index. Korea and Japan ranked the lowest. (The PPP adjustment refers to using the actual purchasing power parity, instead of the foreign exchange rates, for making international comparison of GDP

This chapter is revised/updated from Ng (2002).

This chapter may have touched on some sensitive issues. However, I am myself an East-Asian by birth, education, and culture. Thus, I hope that the chapter will be taken as a self-examination aiming at improvement rather than as a criticism by an outsider.

or GNP per capita. The PPP-adjusted ones reflect more the actual purchasing power, not inflated/deflated by possibly excessively high/low foreign exchange values of the currency of the country concerned.)

For recent surveys, in all the 2018, 2019 and 2020 World Happiness Reports, none of the top twenty countries in happiness ranking are East-Asian. (Taiwan narrowly made the top 19th for the 2021 Report.) At the time of writing, for the latest 2020 Report (based on data over 2017–2019), Singapore (which has a per-capita PPP-adjusted GDP higher than that of the U.S.) came second (to Taiwan, which ranks number 25 worldwide) in the Asian countries/regions in happiness score; it ranked only at 31 (but climbing from 34 in the previous year) out of 153 countries in the world with data. Malaysia (82) and Mainland China (94) both ranked well below the mid-point of the 153 countries. Despite its economic stagnation, Japan (62) ranked much higher than before the three 'lost decades' (For the 2021 report based on the 2020 scores, Japan jumped further to number 40 in the ranking.)

In fact, this 'rise of Japan' in happiness despite economic stagnation may be described as a sister paradox, the paradox of happy stagnation, in comparison to the well-known Easterlin's (1974, 2017) paradox of unhappy growth (discussed in several places earlier). Over the three decades of economic stagnation, the average working hours in Japan also decreased significantly while its happiness level climbed from second last (above only Korea; see Cummins 1998) to just below average (Diener 2000), and then above average (Leigh and Wolfers 2006), and finally to the respectable 62th and 40th out of 153 countries in the World Happiness Reports 2020 and 2021 respectively, as mentioned above. Perhaps people in Japan spent too much time working during their heyday of high economic growth, and then realized their mistake and work less?

This should make us pause to reflect on some fundamental issues like the ultimate ends, the worth, and the costs of economic growth[1]; the reasons for the relative failure of the East Asians in achieving happiness despite their economic success; the implications on ways to increase happiness and for public policies. Due to the unevenness of the level of economic progress, this chapter is more relevant for the more developed parts of East Asia. (On the precise meaning of happiness, the argument that it is the appropriate ultimate objective, and related issues, see Chaps. 1 and 5.)

With the rapid growth in East Asia, researchers have discussed the (largely positive) effects of Confucianism on economic growth. However, the East-Asian happiness gap and its possible relation to the Confucian cultures have been largely neglected. I am quite aware that this is a sensitive area. I also do not have enough expertise in the area to give a complete discussion. However, since happiness is the most important and the ultimate objective in life, it is important to discuss this in the open so that perhaps suitable remedies may be forthcoming if more people become interested.

---

[1] For some forerunners discussing the welfare costs of economic growth by well-known economists, see Mishan (1969/1993) and Scitovsky (1976/1992).

The low ranking of East Asian countries in happiness is consistent with some other measures. For example, according to the Durex report in 2014 (http://library.northernlight.com/FB20001017290000041.html), the satisfaction in sex life, Japan topped the least satisfaction list by a wide margin. Other countries/regions with low sex satisfaction include Hong Kong and Singapore. The average age of first sex (so-called 'loss of virginity') is also highest in Asia (21.8 years old) in contrast to the lowest continent's (South America) Figure of 17.4.

An older Durex survey of 18 thousand adults in 27 countries and regions reported in the mass media world-wide on 17–18 October 2000, Japan also had the lowest average number of sex over a year, 37, far behind the second lowest (Malaysia) of 62 and the low figures for other East-Asian regions (Mainland China 69, Taiwan 78, Hong Kong 84). In comparison, the overall average of 96 is exceeded by, among others, India (95), Brazil (113) and U.S. (132, the top figure). (Document available at http://library.northernlight.com/FB20001017290000041.html.) More recent figures (Beauchamp 2015) show a similar pattern: The lowest figure of 45 times for Japan is far below the second lowest Figure of 73 for Singapore, and less than one third that of the highest 138 times of Greece. The figures of 78 for Hong Kong, 88 for Taiwan, 96 for Mainland China are all within the lowest ten worldwide.

Japan is also the only country in the world where a higher percentage of people report being dissatisfied with their sex lives than satisfied. The least satisfied (in sex) countries/regions are, in descending order: Japan, France, Hong Kong, Singapore, Thailand. 'It's not surprising that the Japanese are having infrequent, unsatisfying sex. For years, Japan reported some of the longest average working hours in the world. [But lower hours in recent years; see above.] In and of itself, this makes sex less likely … Asian countries have a much higher mean age of virginity loss than nations basically everywhere else.' (Beauchamp 2015). According to Chatsbin (http://chartsbin.com/view/xxj), the top countries/regions of highest age in having first sex are all Asian (in descending order with ages in brackets): Malaysia (23), India (22.9), Singapore (22.8), China (22.1), Thailand (20.5), Hong Kong (20.2), Vietnam (19.7), in comparison to the lowest figure of 15.6 years old in Iceland.

Scholars in Asia also agree that Confucianism has the tendency to promote abstinence. The three traditionally influential religions/beliefs of Confucianism, Daoism, and Buddhism in China and other East Asian countries 'all promote the reduction of material desire to pursue happiness/well-being' (Gao et al. 2010, p.1043). What we want to discuss next is the reasons for the East-Asian happiness gap, especially for given levels (and growth rates) of per-capita income and education level (See Veenhoven 2014; Ngoo et al. 2015; Kim 2018 for further evidence on this gap; Lim et al. 2020 on some empirical analysis.)

13.2 Some Reflections

I do not profess to have the complete explanation and answers. However, since I believe that, ultimately, happiness is the most, if not the only, important thing, I wish to venture some reflections. Incomplete and immature as they may be, these bricks may still serve to attract jades.

13.2.1 Why Still the Rat-Race for Money?

If happiness is the ultimate objective and more incomes no longer increase happiness, why do people still engage in the rat race for making more and more money? This may be explained by: the environmental disruption effects, relative-income/consumption effects (emphasized by researchers from Easterlin 1974 to Rojas 2019), the inadequate recognition of adaptation effects, and the irrational materialistic bias, as also discussed in the previous chapters (Chap. 7 in particular). To some extent, it is individually rational to make more money, as higher incomes still contribute marginally to happiness through the importance of relative standing. At the social level, the relative-income effects between individuals cancel each other to leave no effect overall. In addition, the environmental disruption effects of higher production and consumption may really make people worse off. We may have welfare-reducing growth but for the positive effects of the advancement in knowledge. (On welfare-reducing growth despite individual and government optimization, see Ng 2003.) After the survival and moderate comfort levels (wen bao 温飽 and xiao kang 小康), since the positive effect is really very small in terms of long-term real happiness, it is still irrational even at the individual level to sacrifice things more important for happiness such as family, friends, health, and even safety and freedom in order to make more money as many people obviously do, including myself to some extent. But why do people have such irrational preferences? To a large extent, this may be explained by our accumulation instinct and instinct for competition for relative standing (nature) and the effects of the omnipresent advertising and peer influence in our commercial society (nurture). (See Ng 2003 for more details.)

13.2.2 The East Asian Happiness Gap: Its Causes

Even if high incomes no longer increase happiness, perhaps, dynamically, we need rising incomes just to sustain happiness at an unchanged level, the so-called 'hedonic treadmill'. The East Asians have not only high income levels but also high rates of growth in incomes. On these counts, they should be happier than others. Despite these, they are less happy than others. This may be called the East Asian happiness gap. Since our measures of happiness are not foolproof, we cannot be completely confident of the existence of such a gap. However, there is sufficient evidence for provisionally accepting the hypothesis of a gap before it is overthrown by more solid evidence.

Some explanations of the East Asian happiness gap are related to the explanation of the rat-race in the previous subsection. First, the higher congestion, pollution, and other forms of environmental disruption caused by high growth in production and consumption, especially in the heavily congested cities and industrial areas may partly explain why the rapid growth in East Asia is not an unmixed blessing, to say the least. These problems also exist in the West, but are more serious in East Asia due to the higher population density and less adequate environmental protection. Some more genuine indicator of progress that take account of congestion and environmental disruption that are largely ignored by the conventional GDP may show that the growth rates are not as spectacular. Certainly at the margin, it is undesirable to poison our air and water to have additional inessential output. The human costs in ill health in many cities are intolerable. In East Asia's major cities, air and water pollution are the sources of many premature deaths, bronchitis, and respiratory symptoms.[2] The severity of smog in Chinese cities, especially in Northern China including Beijing, and especially over late Autumn to Winter, is well known. As reported, while China has made progress cutting smog, the damage to the health of millions of people may already have been done, especially as the population ages, according to a U.S.-based research agency (Stanway 2018). According to the annual State of Global Air Report by the Health Effects Institute, the annual figures of air-pollution related deaths per 100,000 in 2016 are 117 for China and 21 for the U.S., a difference of more than five and a half times (MaCarthy 2018). Also, the under-reporting of such figures is probably more serious in China.

Secondly, the East-Asians are reputed to be highly competitive. This partly explains their economic success. However, the very high degree of competitiveness may be detrimental in achieving happiness both at the individual level and, even more so, at the social level. One important aspect of competitiveness is trying to surpass others. An individual may succeed in surpassing others but for the whole society, an individual on average cannot surpass others. Much effort in achieving relative distinction, if spent on areas without significant external benefits, may thus be largely wasted socially. (Thus, people should compete in areas with external benefits such as contributions to knowledge and society.) Another aspect of competitiveness is not being contented with one's current achievement and wanting to do better. While this may propel progress in objective terms such as production, it is likely to be detrimental to contentment and happiness.[3]

Buddhism, Hinduism, and Taoism are more emphatic on the virtue of contentedness while Confucianism is, at least relative to the previous three, more emphatic on the virtue of achievement. While Buddhism and Taoism are still believed in parts of East Asia, their influence has largely waned, especially relative to the importance of Buddhism and Hinduism in India.

It is true that we need some degree of competitiveness just to survive and a little more to make progress. However, too high a degree of competitiveness may be detrimental to happiness. In fact, one of the reasons the East-Asians have a high degree of

---

[2] On some regional evidence in China, see Yang et al. (2020). On the feasibility and importance of environmental protection, especially using economical ones, see Guo et al. (2020).

[3] On the positive and negative effects of envy and a distinction between malicious and benign envies, see J.C.K. Ng et al. (2020).

subjective competitiveness may be due to the high degree of competitiveness that has existed objectively for many generations. The competitive environment favors those with a high degree of competitiveness which in turn increases the competitiveness of the environment, completing a vicious cycle. However, the cycle is not unchecked as excessive competitiveness also generates detrimental effects.

Thirdly, the educational method and general cultural influence of the East Asians are also highly productive in competitive achievements (especially in formal examinations) but likely detrimental to real creativity and personal and social happiness. According to the 2015 report (the 2019 results are only forthcoming, as of June 19, 2020) of TIMSS (Trends in International Mathematics and Science Study; https://timss.bc.edu/timss2019/index.html), the East-Asian countries/regions (Mainland China not included in the study) lead the world (49 countries tested) in both math and science in student performance, with Singapore (618), Hong Kong (615), Korea (608), Taiwan (597), Japan (593) at the top in math, and with a big gap of 23 points with the next country of Northern Ireland (570); this gap was the same as the 2011 report. In comparison, England scored 546 (just after Northern Ireland) and the U.S. scored 539; the lowest score by Kuwait was 353. The corresponding figures for science are: Singapore (590), Korea (589), Japan (569), Russia (567), Hong Kong (557), Taiwan (555), U.S. (546), England (536), Kuwait (337) [The 2019 results are now available from the site given above, with no substantial changes to the 2015 ones reported here, e.g. in maths, the top five are still the same countries/regions: Singapore (625), Hong Kong (602), Korea (600), Taiwan (599), Japan (593), with the top Singapore pulling ahead further.].

However, commenting on a previous similar report in 2000, Yuan Tzeh Lee (a Nobel laureate and President of Academia Sinica in Taipei) said, 'Most Taiwan students are good in examinations. Their performance in science and mathematics are good at the stage of high school. However, after graduating from high schools, they become exhausted, as if going to retire ... The educational system in Taiwan is very repressive of curious students interested in pursuing creativity. This is very bad.' (My translation back from my Chinese translation of a report in *China Times*, 7 December 2000, p. 7.) At least to a large extent, this remark is also applicable to other East-Asian regions and also with respect to happiness, not just with respect to creativity.[4]

Fourthly and relatedly, East-Asian culture (especially its educational system) is over-emphatic on conformity, order, and the collective interests to the detriment of individualism, freedom, and hence happiness. It is true that individual freedom must not be excessive either, as the welfare of others may be adversely affected by the relentless and unrestricted pursuit of individual freedom. However, while the West may be somewhat over the delicate balance to be too emphatic of individualism in some aspects, the East-Asians are likely to err in the opposite direction by a wider margin. An important explanation of this big difference is probably related to the relative effectiveness of the legal system in the West which can be relied more to

---

[4] See also Qu et al. (2020) on the happiness 'cost of academic focus' on Chinese school children and their parents in America.

control the excess of individual freedom. This means that, with the legal system strengthened (as obviously very successful in regions like Singapore, Taiwan, and Hong Kong, until the recent couple of years in the last one), East-Asians may move towards the direction of freedom and individualism to increase happiness.

Happiness researchers remark: '… in the Latin nations, such as Colombia, there is a tendency to view pleasant emotions as desirable… In contrast, in Confucian cultures, such as China, there tends to be relatively more acceptance of unpleasant emotions and relatively less acceptance of pleasant emotions… In China the ideal level of life satisfaction was considered to be neutrality—neither satisfied nor dissatisfied' (Diener and Suh 1999, pp. 443–4). Eastern researchers also agree on the 'abstinence' (禁慾) tendency of Confucianism. For example, 'in Confucian culture … abstinence is an important factor' (Fu傅佩荣 1989, p. 51; my translation) and 'hedonistic striving for happiness is regarded as unworthy and even shameful' (Lu and Shih 1997, p. 183; see also Fang 1980, p.153.). The three traditionally influential religions/beliefs of Confucianism, Daoism, and Buddhism in China and other East Asian countries, as also mentioned above, 'all promote the reduction of material desire to pursue happiness/well-being' (Gao, et al. 2010, p. 1043. On the effects of societal values on happiness, especially the relationship between income and happiness, see Lim et al. 2019). How can one enjoy life happily if one is brought up to be adverse to pleasant feelings? (One indication of the abstinence tendency is the high average ages of first time in having sex for East-Asian countries/regions mentioned in Sect. 13.1)

Fifthly, East-Asian culture is too emphatic on appearance, on not losing face and less on the real content and true feelings. The importance of 'face' (面子; mian4 zi3; the numbers here refer to the tones) is well-known. The emphasis on outward appearance in contrast to inner content may be 'spotted' (可窥一斑) in the example of the styles of buildings. The Temple of Heaven (天壇) in Beijing is extremely impressive looking from outside but rather ordinary inside. Most Western churches look rather dull from outside but are well furnished and decorated inside. When my father (born and grew up in China and lived in Malaysia for decades) first saw our flat/apartment (rented) in Australia, he thought that the building (brick-veneered) looked unfinished. When he went inside, he found it very comfortably furnished. Many flats in East Asia have a very small bathroom and kitchen but relatively large 'visitors hall' (客厅) which is known in the West as the lounge room or living room. This difference in the naming of the same room also betrays the difference in emphasis between the East (to impress the visitors) and the West (for the comfort of the family). To what extent is this a reflection of more visitors rather than a difference in emphasis remains to be investigated.

For another example, when advising their children regarding marriage, most Western parents put happiness first. In contrast, many East-Asian parents emphasize the family backgrounds (门当户对) and other objective aspects. It is more important to them (at least relative to people of the West) for the marriage to look good in appearance than for the children to actually have a happy life.

Of course, happiness is also affected by biological factors. However, since they are less amenable to policy influence (except in the future when genetic engineering may be safely used), they are not emphasized here. (On the use of brain stimulation for pleasure and genetic engineering for our own transformation, see Chap. 12 above.)

While cultural differences are important, their role must not be exaggerated. Cultural differences do make a difference as to what factors may affect happiness (e.g. Christopher 1999) but not with respect to the concept and ultimate value of happiness as such. Moreover, there are largely universal factors determined by biology. Thus, Maslow's (1943, 1954/1970a/1987) need-gratification theory of well-being is largely universal (Sect. 10.1 above). Also, I believe that, at the ultimate level, happiness as the rational end (Chap. 5 above) is culturally independent. It may be thought that my personal views on happiness are largely due to the influence of Western culture. However, I can vouch that I was brought up in largely Eastern influence, attending only Chinese schools and university in Malaysia and Singapore before my time of post-graduate study. Even now, my cultural influences are more Chinese than Western. For example, I still read most non-economics books and magazines in Chinese and listen mostly to Chinese music. I can read and write in Chinese almost twice as fast as in English.

Some researchers exaggerate the cultural difference. For example, Lu and Shih (1997, p. 181/2) mention that 'the word happiness did not appear in the Chinese language until recently', suggesting that the concept of happiness is alien to the Chinese people until recently. This is certainly very misleading. It may be true that the modern *phrase* for happiness in Chinese (快乐; kuai4 le4) appeared only recently. However, the ancient *words* for happiness in Chinese (either kuai4 or le4) appeared from time immemorial. For example, le4 appeared in such ancient expressions as 'Friends coming from afar, am I not happy?' (有朋自远方来, 不亦乐乎?) and '[I am] so happy, no more thought of Shu' (乐不思蜀), with the clear meaning of happiness. I suggest that such primitive concepts as happiness are universal and should exist in all cultures from time immemorial, probably not long after the evolution of *homo sapiens*, if not earlier; likely advanced animals also have such concepts, even if they may not be able to verbalize them.

13.3 Some Implications

As the study of happiness has made much progress (e.g. including a journal specializing on the study of happiness, the *Journal of Happiness Study* having produced 22 volumes with many issues each), the importance of happiness and the preliminary results on the failure of higher income/consumption to increase happiness imply that a lot more resources should be used for happiness study. How could the measures of happiness be made more reliable and comparable interpersonally? (Chap. 6 above.) Does the East-Asian happiness gap really exist? Are people of East-Asian origin but living in the West also less happy? How could happiness be increased? Such questions are very important but very much under-researched.

Despite the failure of higher incomes to increase happiness, I continue to believe in the usefulness of economic growth. However, the direction of growth has to be appropriate. First, the protection of environmental quality has to be a top priority. We want clean growth, not dirty growth. Secondly, we want growth that can really increase our happiness. This includes less on largely mutually canceling competitive private consumption and more on areas of public spending that can really increase our welfare. Among others, this includes more public funding for research to find out more. The desirability of higher public spending applies to many other areas including environmental protection, public health, education, and research (More in Chaps. 14 and 15).

Another implication is the need, both at the individual and the social level, to put more emphasis on things that are much more important to happiness than money, including health, relationships, and spiritual fulfillment, as discussed in other chapters of this book. In particular, for the developed parts of East Asia, more reflections on the East-Asian happiness gap are needed. Perhaps it is desirable to realize more about the illusions of the irrational accumulation instinct, to resist more the temptations created by the omnipresent commercial advertising, to reduce our competitive nature, to divert competition from consumption to social contributions, and to make *less* money in order to enjoy life more. East-Asians may not only achieve more happiness this way, but also, by reducing and redirecting their lopsided growth, contribute to a better global environment. (This touches on the issue of international cooperation to address the problem of international competition, a negative-sum game, on which see Ng and Liu 2003.)

However, there are still large parts of East Asia where the majority of people are still very poor by any standard and where economic growth will likely increase the happiness of people significantly. For purely economic development, more emphasis to the development of such areas, including the western regions of China, may be desirable. For the more developed areas of East Asia, factors really important for happiness such as public health, the environment, and above all, the advance in science, technology and knowledge in general, are more important than the purely economic factors such as GDP.

References

BEAUCHAMP, Zack (2015). *6 maps and charts that explain sex around the world*, https://www.vox.com/2014/5/7/5662608/in-different-area-codesdownloaded on 12 July 2019

CHRISTOPHER, John C. (1999). Situating psychological well-being: Exploring the cultural roots of its theory and research. Journal of Counseling & Development, 77(2): 141–152.

CUMMINS, Robert A. (1998). The second approximation to an international standard for life satisfaction. Social Indicators Research, 43: 307–344.

DIENER, Ed (2000). Subjective well-being: the science of happiness and a proposal for a national index. American Psychologist, 55: 34–43.

DIENER, Ed & SUH, Eunkook (1999).National differences in subjective well-being. Chapter 22 in KAHNEMAN, D., DIENER, E. & SCHWARZ, N. *Well-being: The foundations of hedonic psychology* (pp. 434–450). New York, NY, US: Russell Sage Foundation.

FANG, Dong-Mei (方東美 1980). <<中國人生哲學>> (*Chinese Philosophy of Life*), 台北: 黎明出版社(Taipei: Li-Ming).

FU, Pei-rong傅佩荣 (1989).*儒家與現代人生(Confucianism and Modern Life)*, 台北: 業強出版社 (Taipei: Ye Qiang).
GAO, Liang, et al. (2010). The differences in happiness/well-being between China and the West. 高良、郑雪&严标宾 (2010). 幸福感的中西差异: 自我建构的视角.《心理科学进展》, 18(07): 1041–45.
GUO, S., WANG, W. & ZHANG, M. (2020). Exploring the impact of environmental regulations on happiness: new evidence from China. Environmental Science and Pollution Research, 27: 19484–19501. DOI: https://doi.org/10.1007/s11356-020-08508-7
KIM, Donghwan (2018). Cross-national pattern of happiness: Do higher education and less urbanization degrade happiness? Applied Research in Quality of Life, 13(1), 21–35.
LEIGH, A. & WOLFERS, J. (2006). Happiness and the human development index: Australia is not a paradox. Australian Economic Review, 39(2), 176–184.
LIM, Hock-Eam, SHAW, D., LIAO, P. et al. (2020). The effects of income on happiness in East and South Asia: Societal values matter?. Journal of Happiness Studies 21, 391–415. https://doi.org/10.1007/s10902-019-00088-9
LU, Lau & SHIH, Jian Bin (1997). Sources of happiness: A qualitative approach. Journal of Social Psychology, 137: 181–187.
MASLOW, A. H. (1943). A theory of human motivation. Psychological Review, 50(4), 370–396.
MASLOW, Abraham H. (1954/1970a/1987). *Motivation and Personality*. New York: Harper & Row/ Delhi, India: Pearson Education.
MISHAN, Ezra J. (1969/1993), *The Costs of Economic Growth*, London: Weidenfeld & Nicolson.
NG, J.C.K., AU, A.K.Y., WONG, H.S.M. *et al.* (2020). Does Dispositional Envy Make You Flourish More (or Less) in Life? An Examination of Its Longitudinal Impact and Mediating Mechanisms Among Adolescents and Young Adults. *Journal of Happiness Studies*. https://doi.org/10.1007/s10902-020-00265-1
NG, Yew-Kwang. (2002). The East-Asian happiness gap. *Pacific Economic Review*, 7(1), 51–63.
NG, Yew-Kwang & LIU, Po-Ting (2003). Global environmental protection – solving the international public-good problem by empowering the United Nations through cooperation with WTO. International Journal of Global Environmental Issues, 3(4): 409–417.
NGOO, Yee Ting, TEY, Nai Peng & TAN, Eu Chye (2015). Determinants of life satisfaction in Asia. Social Indicators Research, 124(1):141–156.
QU, Y., YANG, B. & TELZER, E.H. (2020). The cost of academic focus: Daily school problems and biopsychological adjustment in Chinese American families. J Youth Adolescence 49, 1631–1644. https://doi.org/10.1007/s10964-020-01255-5
ROJAS, Mariano (Ed.) (2019). *The Economics of Happiness: How the Easterlin Paradox Transformed Our Understanding of Well-Being and Progress*, Springer.
SCITOVSKY, Tibor (1976/1992), *The Joyless Economy*, New York: Oxford University Press.
STANWAY, D. (2018). *China cuts smog but health damage already done: study*. Reuters, April 17, 2018.
VEENHOVEN, R. (2014). *World Database of Happiness*. Available from: http://worlddatabaseofhappiness.eur.nl
YANG, X., GENG, L. & ZHOU, K. (2020). Environmental pollution, income growth, and subjective well-being: regional and individual evidence from China. Environmental Science and Pollution Research. https://doi.org/10.1007/s11356-020-09678-0.

Open Access This chapter is licensed under the terms of the Creative Commons Attribution 4.0 International License (http://creativecommons.org/licenses/by/4.0/), which permits use, sharing, adaptation, distribution and reproduction in any medium or format, as long as you give appropriate credit to the original author(s) and the source, provide a link to the Creative Commons license and indicate if changes were made.

The images or other third party material in this chapter are included in the chapter's Creative Commons license, unless indicated otherwise in a credit line to the material. If material is not included in the chapter's Creative Commons license and your intended use is not permitted by statutory regulation or exceeds the permitted use, you will need to obtain permission directly from the copyright holder.

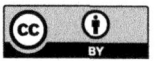

Chapter 14
Implications for Public Policy

Abstract The failure of higher private consumption to increase happiness significantly due to environmental disruption, relative competition, adaptation, our materialistic bias, etc. are relevant for public policy, especially in making higher public spending in the right areas like environmental protection, research, poverty elimination, etc. more welfare-improving than a 'big society, small government'. Some soft paternalistic measures such as nudging people to save adequately for old age may also be needed in the widespread presence of imperfect rationality and foresight.

The policy implications of findings in happiness studies partly depend on our understanding of the reasons for these findings. Most economists focus on the important role of relative standing. Thus, in his seminal paper, Easterlin (1974) uses it to explain the failure of happiness to increase. Once over the subsistence level, happiness depends more on relative than absolute levels of incomes, consumption, or other objective variables.[1] In fact, Knight et al. (2013) show that relative income was at least twice as important for individual happiness as absolute income, even in rural China where people were barely above the subsistence level. Studies in the West show less dramatic results but still have relative incomes at least half as important as absolute incomes. Frank (1999), Ireland (1998), and others correctly draw the conclusion that this implies very high corrective taxes on incomes (Cf. Luo et al. 2018). In fact, all of the income taxes of most countries could be justified as corrective taxes on the relative competition effects alone. If we add the very substantial environmental costs of most production and consumption, general taxation is likely to be below its optimally efficient level. Rather than imposing excess burdens or distortionary costs, taxes are corrective and this efficiency gain could be increased by increasing tax rates! This would stand traditional public economics on this aspect on its head! (Yan et al. 2021.)

Another important factor accounting for the findings in happiness that appear to be inconsistent with traditional presumption in economics is the importance of

---

[1] For another explanation based on the role of cultural values, see Ahuvia (2002).

adaptation effects (people get used to their standard of living) and the underestimation of these effects by most if not all people.[2] There are also a host of other results indicating that individuals are far from being perfectly rational. Moreover, this imperfection does not just cause random biases on either side. Rather, partly due to the nature of accumulation instinct and partly to nurture (peer pressure and commercial advertising), there is a consistent bias towards excessive materialism (Ng 2003). A distinction between utility (representing preference) and welfare (happiness) is thus necessary (Chap. 2). Traditional welfare economics and cost–benefit analysis are based on individual preferences or willingness to pay. When individual preference and welfare systematically diverge, adjustments may be necessary even in the absence of external effects.

A cost–benefit analysis aiming to maximize happiness (or welfare; the two terms are used interchangeably) may be quite different from one aiming at net-income or even preference maximization (including Pareto optimality in the sense of preference). For example, if certain protection measure is shown to cost the economy more than the total wages of the protected workers, most economists regard this as more than conclusive proof that the measure is inefficient. However, while this is inefficient in terms of income maximization, it needs not be inefficient in terms of happiness maximization. The protective measure may well still be inefficient in happiness terms if unemployment will only increase very temporarily without the measure. If displaced workers could get alternative jobs quickly, no protection is usually the best choice. However, if prolonged unemployment will be involved, it may be worth spending more than the total wages to protect the jobs. This is so because of two results in happiness studies: 1. Unemployment causes a lot of unhappiness which is ways beyond the mere losses in incomes (Winkelmann and Winkelmann 1998; see also Sect. 10.3); 2. At least for rich countries, more incomes no longer contribute to happiness at the social level in the long run (Chap. 7). It may thus make sense to spend a lot of money at negligible marginal happiness to protect jobs that are important for happiness. Economists' case against protection has to rest more with the working of the market to make unemployment temporary. This also implies the higher importance of job search or transition assistance.

Consider issues like accidents/risk/security, health care, and the value of life. Modern economics has replaced incomes-based analysis with willingness-to-pay or preference-based analysis. If we ignore possible concern for others, ignorance and irrational preferences, individual preference and welfare coincide and analysis based on preference and that based on welfare are equivalent at the individual level. At the social level, we then only have to take into account external effects and issues of equality that economists are already familiar with. However, recent results in happiness studies and behavioural economics suggest that individual choices often involve imperfect information and/or imperfect rationality and this is so especially for choices involving the future and changes in small probabilities. In combination with the basis of excessive materialism/consumerism mentioned above, this may make

---

[2] See Clark et al. (2008) for a survey; I discussed the happiness implications of aspiration and adaptation in Ng (1978) and Ng and Wang (1993).

14 Implications for Public Policy

people engage in excessive competition/consumption (to the detriment of health and family life), under-save for old age (making compulsory superannuation possibly sensible and actually practised in many countries), and also a host of other welfare-reducing activities not warranted even at the individual level (before counting the additional external costs through the environmental and relative-income effects). Thus, asking people's willingness to pay for a marginal increase in safety or a slight reduction in the risk of a fatal accident may not give reliable values of life in the sense of true expected welfare maximization.

On the one hand, such figures may be under-reported due to people's pressure for present consumption and hence under-rating the willingness to pay for safety. On the other hand, these figures may be over-reported due to the innate irrational fear of death (which has clear selection value but may be inconsistent with welfare maximization). Thus, it is desirable to supplement the willingness-to-pay studies with happiness studies. For expected welfare maximization,[3] the value of life should equal the total happiness of remaining life divided by the true happiness value of a marginal dollar. Since this latter value is likely to be very low (if still positive) even just taking into account the adaptation effect alone, the correct value of life may be very large even at the individual level. At the social level, this is even more so, as the true happiness value of a marginal dollar has to be further discounted by environmental effects and the mutually offsetting relative-income effects. This may partly explain the very large sums of money some decision makers at the social level are willing to spend to improve safety that most economists regard as many times beyond the efficient levels. While there may be some efficiency problems at the public decision-making level, it may also be the case that economists should revise their analysis to be more consistent with welfare maximization.

A particular area where very substantial adjustments are necessary is public spending. Since government spending on public goods has to be financed from taxation and government spending may involve some unavoidable inefficiency, most economists emphasize the excess burden of taxation and are in favour of lowering government spending. Their favorite slogan is: Big society, small government. This position ignores the probably greater inefficiency of private production and consumption due to unaccounted-for environmental costs and the mutually cancelling effects (at the social level) of competition for relative standing. In addition, if additional private consumption no longer contributes to happiness at the social level, even if the monetary costs of public spending are very high, but the ultimate happiness costs may be zero. Thus, provided that the relevant items of public spending do contribute to happiness ultimately, they may still be worth the high costs and some inefficiency in public spending. In addition, there are also arguments (Kaplow 1996; Ng 2000) that, even if we ignore these factors, the spending side tends to produce offsetting effects to the excess burden on the taxation side, as discussed in the next chapter.

If individual choices are subject to high degrees of informational imperfection and irrationality, does that mean that central planning is better than the market economy?

---

[3] For the argument that this is the appropriate objective in the presence of risk/uncertainty, see Ng (1984).

Our experience gives a clear and resounding 'No!'. Soviet Union, Eastern European countries, and China all adopted central planning without success. Central planners are also subject to imperfections in knowledge, rationality, and motivation. Much government interventions especially nationalization in Western countries also do not give an encouraging experience. We should not go back to central planning and use inappropriate government intervention. These paternalistic measures not only usually less efficient than the imperfect private market, they also temper with individual freedom excessively. Nevertheless, while the government should not be too paternalistic, some milder degree of so-called 'soft paternalism' or libertarian paternalism may work to revise the mistakes of imperfect private decisions. This is advocated by, among others, Richard Thaler (Nobel laureate in economics in 2017) and his collaborator Cass Sustein, including in their joint book called *Nudge* (Thaler and Sustein 2009; updated edition). See also: Camerer et al. (2003), Lambert (2017); for criticism/evaluation of soft paternalism, see: Qizilbash (2012), Rebonato (2014), Fumagalli (2016), Epstein (2018); for welfare-improving measures beyond soft paternalism, see Bhargave and Loewenstein (2015).

One very successful soft-paternalistic policy is nudging people to have more savings. Under saving for retirement while in prime working ages is an important problem in many Western countries. In the U.S. Congress, the rightist conservatives and the leftist liberals united to push through the policy of 'Save more tomorrow'. If you ask people to save more right now, resistance is very high. Instead, people are requested to agree now that, when their salaries increase next, they will save more a proportion of the increase. This does not require people to cut down consumption and hence wins much higher rates of acceptance. Apart from the U.S., other countries including the U.K. and South Korea also accept some soft-paternalistic policies.

Another mild policy of restriction is for countries/states where legal gambling is allowed, including Singapore and some states in the U.S., to allow people to apply for restricting themselves or family members from entering casinos. In the State of Michigan in the U.S., the person who first applied for such a restriction on himself was also the first to be arrested for violating that restriction. After signing to restrict himself, he could not control himself and sneaked into a casino to play blackjack. After being discovered, he was not only fined but his winning of more than a thousand U.S. dollars was also confiscated.

Why do people restrict themselves? Studies show that emotion and reasoning are handled in different parts in our brain. While one is calmly reasoning, one may realize that gambling is no good for oneself. However, when one is emotionally attracted, reasoning may not be able to control your emotion.

If people have demand for restricting themselves, why could such restriction not be supplied by the market? This is so because, in the absence of the power of enforcement by the government, the emotional self will cancel the restriction by the rational self. For example, in the eighteenth century, the romantic poet Samuel Taylor Coleridge of the U.K. employed workers to prevent him to go into opium-smoking houses. However, when he wanted to get in, he would warn the workers that, if they prevented him, he would call the police to arrest them.

Due to the widespread existence of laziness, procrastination, vulnerability to temptations, and many other reasons of imperfect rationality, problems like obesity, alcohol poisoning, inadequate savings, etc. are prevalent. Thus, if excessively illiberal policies are avoided, some soft-paternalistic measures may be considered to help people to become healthier and happier. One simple policy is to impose much higher taxes on those demerit goods like cigarettes, soft drinks and candies to reduce their consumption. Apart from this consumption reduction effects, the extra revenues generated could be used for poverty reduction and environmental protection.

In the light of recent results in happiness studies, Layard (2005) has convincingly argued for the need to rethink public policy with respect to many areas including work-life balance, family life, helping the poor, eliminating high unemployment, mental illness, and community life. Here, I wish to mention a couple of areas of public spending that are more likely to increase happiness than private competitive spending.

First, in the light of the threatening effects of climate change and other environmental disruption, public actions in controlling pollution both in the form of taxing external costs and in abatement spending will likely be necessary to protect our future. Economists are familiar with the desirability in principle of taxing external effects in accordance to the damages inflicted. However, for environmental disruption that affects the long future, it is difficult if not impractical to estimate. Even if this is so, for most cases where some abatement is desirable (true for most serious environmental problems including climate change), it is desirable to tax disruption at least at the marginal cost of abatement (which is easier to estimate than the marginal damage of disruption). Such a tax will normally yield total revenue in excess of the optimal amount of abatement spending (Ng 2004). However, due to the global nature of some if not a large part of environmental disruption, international cooperation will likely be necessary. (On ways to foster international cooperation and compliance, see Ng and Liu 2003.)

If we proceed along an environmentally responsible path of growth, our great grandchildren in a century will have a real per capita income 5 to 6 times higher than our level now. Is it worth the risk of environmental disaster to disregard environmental protection now to try to grow a little faster? If this faster growth could be sustained, our great grandchildren would enjoy a real per capita income 7 to 8 times (instead of 5–6 times) higher than our level now. However, they may live in an environmentally horrible world or may well not have a chance to be born at all! The correct choice is obvious.

Easterly (1999) shows that, with economic growth, while some quality-of-life indicators increase, others decrease. Rather, it is the advance in knowledge at the world level that is more positively associated with higher values of quality-of-life indicators. In addition, as knowledge is largely a global public good with long-term benefits, it is likely to be well under-supplied. Thus, public investment in education and research to promote the advance of knowledge will most certainly yield very high benefits. I also support Layard's (2005, Chap.13) endorsement of the *appropriate* use of drugs to promote happiness.[4] However, brain stimulation and genetic engineering provide far more potential, as discussed in Chap. 12. Especially for those with some understanding of economics, the case for higher public spending is pursued at a deeper level in the next chapter, taking account of the argument of Kaplow, a well-accomplished economist of the Harvard Law School.

References

AHUVIA, A. C. (2002). Individualism/collectivism and cultures of happiness: A theoretical conjecture on the relationship between consumption, culture and subjective well-being at the national level. *Journal of Happiness Studies, 3*, 23–36. https://doi.org/10.1023/A:1015682121103

BHARGAVE, S. & LOEWENSTEIN, G. (2015). Behavioral economics and public policy 102: Beyond nudging. *American Economic Review, Papers & Proceedings, 105*(5), 396–401.

CAMERER, C., ISSACHAROFF, S., LOEWENSTEIN, G., O'DONAGHUE, T. & RABIN, M. (2003). Regulation for conservatives: Behavioral economics and the case for "asymmetric paternalism." *University of Pennsylvania Law Review, 151*, 1211–1254.

CLARK, A. E., FRIJTERS, P. & SHIELDS, M. A. (2008). Relative income, happiness, and utility: An explanation for the Easterlin paradox and other puzzles. *Journal of Economic Literature, 46*(1), 95–144.

EASTERLY, William. (1999). Life during growth. *Journal of Economic Growth, 4*(3), 239–276. https://doi.org/10.1023/A:1009882702130

EPSTEIN, Richard A. (2018). The Dangerous allure of libertarian paternalism. *Review of Behavioral Economics, 5*(3–4), 389–416.

FRANK, R. H. (1999). *Luxury Fever: Why Money Fails to Satisfy in an Era of Excess.* Free Press.

FUMAGALLI, R. (2016). Decision sciences and the new case for paternalism: Three welfare-related justificatory challenges. *Soc Choice Welf, 47*, 459–480. https://doi.org/10.1007/s00355-016-0972-1

IRELAND, Norman J. (1998). Status-seeking, income taxation and efficiency. *Journal of Public Economics., 70*, 99–113.

KAPLOW, Louis. (1996). The optimal supply of public goods and the distortionary cost of taxation. *National Tax Journal, 49*(4), 513–533.

LAMBERT, Thomas A. (2017). Symposium: Evaluating Nudge: A Decade of Libertarian Paternalism: Foreward: From Gadfly to Nudge: The Genesis of Libertarian Paternalism, *Missouri Law Review.* 82, Available at: https://scholarship.law.missouri.edu/mlr/vol82/iss3/5

LAYARD, Richard (2005). *Happiness: Lessons from a New Science.* Penguin.

LUO, Yangmei, WANG, Tong, and HUANG, Xiting. (2018). Which types of income matter most for well-being in China: Absolute, relative or income aspirations? *International Journal of Psychology, 53*(3), 218–222.

NG, Yew-Kwang. (1978). Economic growth and social welfare: The need for a complete study of happiness. *Kyklos*, 575–587. *Reprinted in Easterlin, 2002, 66–77.*

NG, Yew-Kwang. (1984). Expected subjective utility: Is the Neumann-Morgenstern utility the same as the neoclassical's? *Social Choice and Welfare, 1*(3), 177–186.

NG, Yew-Kwang. (2000). *Efficiency, Equality, and Public Policy: With a Case for Higher Public Spending.* Macmillan.

---

[4] 'Ironically, what will in the end defeat the bad drugs, especially heroin and cocaine, will be the new medical drugs that work better than they do. These new drugs will be safer and non-addictive. Side by side with cognitive therapies, they will enable people whose natures are rough or whose lives have been tough to become happier people' (Layard 2005, p. 221).

References

NG, Yew-Kwang. (2003). From preference to happiness: Towards a more complete welfare economics", *Social Choice and* Welfare, 20: 307–350.

NG, Yew-Kwang. (2004). Optimal environmental charges/taxes: Easy to estimate and surplus-yielding. *Environmental and Resource Economics, 28*(4), 395–408.

NG, Yew-Kwang & LIU, Po-Ting. (2003). Global environmental protection – solving the international public-good problem by empowering the United Nations through cooperation with WTO. *International Journal of Global Environmental Issues, 3*(4), 409–417.

NG, Yew-Kwang & WANG, Jianguo. (1993). Relative income, aspiration, environmental quality, individual and political myopia: Why may the rat-race for material growth be welfare reducing? *Mathematical Social Sciences, 26*, 3–23.

QIZILBASH, Mozaffar. (2012). Informed desire and the ambitions of libertarian paternalism. *Social Choice and Welfare, 38*, 647–658. https://doi.org/10.1007/s00355-011-0620-8

REBONATO, R. A. (2014). Critical assessment of libertarian paternalism. *Journal of Consumer Policy, 37*, 357–396. https://doi.org/10.1007/s10603-014-9265-1

THALER, Richard H. & SUNSTEIN. Cass R. (2009). (updated edition). *Nudge: Improving Decisions about Health, Wealth, and Happiness*. New York: Penguin.

WINKELMANN, Liliana & WINKELMANN, Rainer. (1998). Why are the unemployed so unhappy? *Economica, 65*, 1–15.

YAN, Eric, FENG, Qu & NG, Y.-K. (2021). Do we need Ramsey taxation? Our existing taxes are largely corrective. *Economic Modelling*, accepted.

Open Access This chapter is licensed under the terms of the Creative Commons Attribution 4.0 International License (http://creativecommons.org/licenses/by/4.0/), which permits use, sharing, adaptation, distribution and reproduction in any medium or format, as long as you give appropriate credit to the original author(s) and the source, provide a link to the Creative Commons license and indicate if changes were made.

The images or other third party material in this chapter are included in the chapter's Creative Commons license, unless indicated otherwise in a credit line to the material. If material is not included in the chapter's Creative Commons license and your intended use is not permitted by statutory regulation or exceeds the permitted use, you will need to obtain permission directly from the copyright holder.

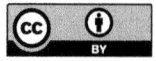

Chapter 15
A Case for Higher Public Spending

Abstract Studies by psychologists, sociologists, and economists indicate that increases in incomes beyond a moderate level are not related to happiness nor significantly with the objective quality-of-life indicators (which increase with scientific and technological breakthroughs at the global level). Yet everyone wants more money. This may be explained by environmental disruption, relative-income effects, inadequate recognition of adaptation effects, and the materialistic bias due to our accumulation instinct and advertising. These factors cause a bias towards private consumption, making public spending, especially on research and environmental protection (with their long-term and global public-good nature) well below optimal. This is made worse by economists' emphasis on the excess burden of taxation, ignoring the negative excess burden on the spending side. As Kaplow argues, if taxes are raised in accordance to the benefits of the funded public goods at the respective income levels, no disincentive effects are involved.

We have discussed the failure of private consumption to significantly increase happiness after a rather low level of biological necessity and comfort (Chap. 7) and discussed some reasons and implications in other chapters. These naturally suggest the question whether we may be able to increase happiness more by increasing public spending, at least in the right areas, as also discussed in the previous chapter. However, the global trends in recent decades seem to be against public spending. The whole world is marching towards the right, with the transformation of the Soviet Union and Eastern Europe, the drastic economic reforms in China, and the privatization, liberalization, and (reversing the historical increasing trend) reduction in taxes (with the Trump's tax reduction in December 2017 being a recent important event) and public spending in many Western countries.[1] Much of these changes are applaudable

---

[1] For example, the share of total general government outlays in GDP increased very substantially over many decades to around 34% in the mid 1980's (1985–1987) in the US but then declined to 30.1% in 1999 and projected to decline to 29.4% in 2001. The corresponding figures for all OECD countries (Australia in brackets) are: 38.3% (36%) in mid 1980's, 37.8% (32.3%) in 1999, and 36.9% (31.8%). (*Source OECD Economic Outlook* June 2000, p. 270.) The proportions have however recovered somewhat in the last decade or so. Conceptually, there are valid arguments for optimal public spending to increase in real per-capita incomes (Ng 2000b).

and economists may feel proud for partially contributing to these changes. However, this chapter argues that the reduction in public spending, especially in education, research, and environmental protection is counter-productive. Imagine a trebling in your income but without access to computers, television, phones, modern medical facilities, etc., wouldn't your welfare be reduced drastically? This may not be so viewed in the narrow perspective of production and consumption especially in the short run, but is almost certainly so viewed in the wider perspective of welfare (or happiness) in the long run and at the social level. It is well known that public spending has some efficiency problems but the probably much worse inefficiency of private consumption has been largely ignored. This chapter attempts to provide a broader and more balanced picture from an interdisciplinary perspective.

15.1 Economists Overestimate the Costs of Public Spending

For a dollar of public spending, non-economists typically cost it at one dollar. However, economists typically cost it at well in excess of one dollar. An estimate by a well-known economist (Feldstein 1997) puts it at $2.65. Though this is an extreme estimate, on average the economists' estimate is for a dollar of public expenditures to be $1.30, a premium of 30%. Such high estimates of the costs of public spending suggest that public projects should yield very high benefits before they are worthwhile to undertake; a benefit-to-cost ratio of 1.3, instead of one, has to be exceeded. This conception probably partly contributes to the worldwide trend towards cuts in public spending.

The costs of public funds include not only its direct cost (the amount of taxes imposed) but also the costs of administration, compliance, policing, and distortion. While the first three types of costs are substantial, they do not vary significantly with the amount of tax revenue raised. Hence, concentrating on the marginal costs of public spending, economists emphasize the distortionary costs or excess burden of taxation due to the fact that taxes distort the free choices of individuals, especially in discouraging work effort, i.e. the disincentive effects. At least since the time of Pigou (1928), economists have emphasized that the benefits of public goods must exceed their direct costs by an amount sufficient to outweigh the excess burden of taxation. An authoritative modern textbook by a Nobel laureate puts the Pigovian principle this way: 'Since it becomes more costly to obtain public goods when taxation imposes distortions, normally this will imply that the efficient level of public goods is smaller than it would have been with non-distortionary taxation' (Stiglitz 1988, p. 140). It is known that this general rule is subject to qualifications due to the presence of considerations like complementarity/substitutivity between public and private goods (Atkinson and Stiglitz 1980; King 1986; Batina 1990; Wilson 1991; Chang 2000). Specific cases or conditions under which the efficient level of public goods is not affected have also been identified (Christiansen 1981; Boadway and Keen 1993; Konishi 1995, Dahlby 2008, Chang et al. 2016, Burns and Ziliak 2017, Jacobs 2018).

15.1 Economists Overestimate the Costs of Public Spending

In contrast to minor qualifications and special cases, a whole scale onslaught on the Pigou principle is presented by Kaplow (1996). He argues that public goods can be financed without additional distortion by using an adjustment to the income tax that offsets the benefits of the public good. The *'preexisting income tax schedule is adjusted so that, at each income level, the tax change just offsets the benefits from the public good. By construction, an individual's net reward from any level of work effort will be unaltered; any reduction in disposable income due to the tax adjustment is balanced by the benefits from the public good. Because an individuals' after-tax utility as a function of his work effort will thus be unchanged, his choice of work effort – and utility level – will also be unaffected'* (Kaplow 1996, p. 514).

For example, if the benefit of a public good is proportional to the income level of the taxpayers, it may be financed by a (or an increase in) proportional income tax. The proportional income tax itself may involve a disincentive effect. However, the tax plus the public good together involve no disincentive effect. Suppose that, for each $100 earned, $20 have to be taxed. Is not the incentive to earn more income less than the case where one can keep the full $100? This lower incentive may well apply if the tax revenue is thrown into the ocean. However, normally the revenue is used for public spending that the taxpayers value more or at least no less (otherwise the public spending is inefficient even using the benefit/cost ratio of one). Suppose the tax revenue is used for police protection of property whose benefits are roughly proportional to the income level. Then, each individual may in fact has higher incentive to earn the protected $80 than the unprotected $100.

While Kaplow's argument has to be qualified in the presence of tax evasion, heterogeneity of individuals at the same income level, benefits from public goods relating to ability than to income, etc., its main thrust is valid (Ng 2000a). How then do we reconcile Kaplow's argument with the orthodox position of the high costs of public spending? First, Feldstein (1997) obtains his high estimate of $2.65 by including policy-intended effects as unwanted distortions. He emphasises that higher tax rates may not only reduce the supply of labour and capital, but also change the forms in which individuals take their compensation, including more on things that are tax deductible. However, while correctly including tax-induced expenditures on luxurious working conditions, he also includes other tax-deductible items like 'charitable gifts, and health care' as involving distortions. However, these items are what the society/government want to encourage either on the grounds of external benefits (e.g. the prevention of communicable diseases), poverty reduction, and possibly merit wants (though the last ground is more controversial). Provided the extent of tax-deductibility is not excessive, no net distortion is created. Or, the extent of the distortion is offset by the benefits (Ng 2000a).

Secondly, Feldstein's (1997) high estimate ignores the argument of Kaplow (1996). Alternatively stated, while the cost of a dollar of public spending on the revenue side may be much higher than $1, the excess may be largely offset by the positive incentive (or negative disincentive) effects of the spending side. If the benefits of the public spending are not positively correlated with income such that there is no positive incentive effects on the spending side but only disincentive effects on the revenue side, there is a distributional benefit since the rich pay more and the poor pay less (Kaplow 1996; Ng 2000a).

Since high tax rates also encourage tax avoidance and evasion and since some higher benefits of public goods are related to unobservable earning ability than observable income levels, the positive incentive effects on the spending side may not completely offset the distortive effects on the revenue side, making a dollar of public spending still in excess of a dollar taking both sides into account. However, the considerations of the prevalence of environmental costs of most production and consumption, relative competition, the failure of higher private consumption to increase happiness at the social level, as argued in the previous chapters (and Ng 2003; Yan, et al. 2021), suggest that the cost of a dollar of public spending should be significantly reduced (likely to well below one dollar and possibly towards zero) or that the benefits of public spending should be significantly increased from those normally estimated by economists.

The general taxes on income and consumption, though designed mainly for the purpose of revenue raising, may in fact serve as rough counteracting measures to the environmental disruption effects involved. Thus, far from being distortive, taxation may be corrective; instead of imposing positive excess burdens or distortionary costs, taxation may serve to improve efficiency. The relative-income effects also cause a bias in favour of private spending or against public spending. In most estimates, the marginal benefit of private expenditure is likely to be taken to include the absolute-income or intrinsic consumption effects *plus* the internal or direct relative income effect (as these two taken together constitute the worth of private consumption as it appears to each individual), but not to include the negative external or indirect relative income effects. This creates an over-emphasis in favour of private expenditure, leading to a sub-optimal level of public spending (Ng 1987a). Similarly, the materialistic bias and the insufficient recognition of the adaptation effects suggest that the opportunity costs of reducing private consumption due to a higher public spending are not as high as most people believe.

In addition to the above considerations, there is another factor making the cost of public spending lower than normally believed – the existence of burden-free taxes. While most economists realize that corrective taxes on, say, pollution involve negative excess burden or positive efficiency gain, burden-free taxes are regarded as existent only in fairyland. However, there are goods taxes on which create not only no *excess* burden but no burden at all, even ignoring all the considerations above. These are pure diamond goods or goods valued for their exchange values rather their intrinsic consumption effects. People consume or hold these goods to show off their wealth, to use them as stores of value or gifts of value. Cubic zirconia looks exactly like top quality diamond but costs only a tiny fraction of true diamond. But no one gives his fiancée an engagement ring of cubic zirconia. For such goods, it is the value (price times quantity) that enters the utility function of the consumer rather than the quantity, as posited in economic analysis. As prices increase due to higher taxes on these goods, consumers may just spend the same amounts to buy the same values without real losses. The revenues raised are pure gains, suggesting arbitrarily high taxes on them (Ng 1987b). While many goods (most precious metals and stones, top brands of most goods especially conspicuous items like cars and wines) possess various degrees of diamond effect, few if any good is a pure diamond good. Nevertheless, very high taxes on mixed diamond goods are still efficient. Moreover, as consumers may wish to consume the value (pure diamond) aspect of the mixed good so much (such as to show off their wealth) as to incur negative utility on the intrinsic consumption aspect (such as health-threatening excessive drinking), taxes on such mixed diamond goods may actually make consumers better off (being able to show off to the same extent without drinking to excess) (Ng 1993).

15.2 Specific Areas of Deficient Public Spending

In a lucid and compelling book, Frank (1999) detailed the enormous waste of conspicuous private consumption (related to relative-consumption effects discussed above) in the U.S. and discusses specific areas where additional public spending will clearly generate welfare gains far in excess of the opportunity costs. *'A century hence, those who read the history of our time will be puzzled about the arguments we have used in defense of cutting, or refusing to fund, so many clearly useful public programs. They will wonder, for example, why we failed to replace our deteriorating municipal water systems, thereby exposing millions of families to toxic levels of lead, manganese, and other heavy metals. They will not understand why we didn't adopt more stringent air-quality standards, which would have prevented millions of serious illnesses and many thousands of premature deaths; or why we didn't hire more beef inspectors in response to the growing threat from deadly E-coli 0157 bacteria. They will be puzzled by our having spent so little to maintain our streets, highways, and bridges. And it will not be obvious to them why, despite our considerable wealth, we failed to pay enough to attract the best and brightest teachers for our public schools.'* (pp. 253–4). *'A Rand Corporation study ... estimated that every $1 spent on cocaine prevention and treatment programs results in a $7 savings in law-enforcement and health-care expenses. Yet consistently we say we cannot afford these programs'* (p. 62).

The above list can easily be expanded. For example, a few examples may be given to indicate that a lot more research is needed to increase welfare.

- The very topic of the appropriate size of the public sector, regarded by Feldstein (1997) as *the* central public finance question, is much under-researched. For example, few if any researchers relate the important issues of relative income and happiness to this central question. While we have discussed this and other related issues above, a lot more analytical and empirical studies are needed.
- While studies on the effects of specific drugs and ingredients have been done, it seems that a general study tracing the different types of food, drugs, and activities taken by a big enough sample of people (in hundreds of thousands) of different ages and health conditions (not just those hospitalized) over a long period (at least in decades) to discover the desirable and undesirable, short and long-run effects, may be most rewarding. Though the study would be very costly, we would gain

very useful knowledge on many thousands of things simultaneously. An analysis suggests that 'even after taking account of distorted incentives, the potential gains to medical advancement are enormous ... easily justify ... expenditures far above current levels' (Murphy & Robert 2000).

- The stimulation of certain pleasure centres in the brain can relieve acute pain, induce intense pleasure, and promote a sense of well-being without the undesirable health effects of drug addiction and without the effect of diminishing marginal utility. It can also be used as a primer such that someone who had never experienced climax before consistently achieve climax in normal sex after the brain stimulation helped to establish the pathway. This method has been known for nearly seven decades (Olds & Milner 1954). Why has the method not been perfected for common use in order to increase happiness, reduce depression, and solve many social and mental problems? (See Chap. 12 above for more details.)

15.3 Concluding Remarks

From the various factors discussed above, the costs of public spending have been grossly overestimated. While it is desirable to do away with the inefficiencies in public spending if possible, even before this is possible, increases in public spending, especially in education, research, and environmental protection, can still increase our welfare. The recent trend of checking the growth in public spending may be grossly inefficient. In fact, economic growth increases the optimal share of public spending and that, without directly dealing with environmental disruption, economic growth may reduce welfare even if the shares of public spending and environmental protection are being optimized (Ng 2003).

In addition to the above considerations, public spending on research and environmental protection is also likely to be grossly sub-optimal due to its long-term and global public-good nature. Scientific advances and a cleaner environment benefit the whole world for generations to come. Decisions taken by national governments with relatively short time horizons results in sub-optimal spending in these areas even before we consider factors accounting for the overestimation of the costs of public spending discussed above (Sect. 15.1). This suggests the need for international cooperation to increase funding for research and environmental protection. In fact, the relative-income effects at the individual level discussed above also applies to the national level, resulting in international competition for income growth, the bias against public spending and the disregard to environmental degradation. This further strengthens the need for international cooperation. The success of such cooperation partly depends on the widespread appreciation of the interdisciplinary arguments as discussed in this chapter and the rest of this book. (For a framework analysing interdisciplinary factors affecting welfare or happiness, see Ng 2004, Chap. 12.)

References

ATKINSON, A. B. & STIGLITZ, J. E. (1980). *Lectures on Public Economics*. McGraw-Hill.

BATINA, Raymond G. (1990). On the interpretation of the modified Samuelson rule for public goods in static models with heterogeneity. *Journal of Public Economics, 42*, 125–133.

BOADWAY, Robin W. & KEEN, Michael. (1993). Public goods, self-selection and optimal income taxation. *International Economic Review, 34*(3), 463–478.

BURNS, Sarah K. & ZILIAK, James P. (2017). Identifying the elasticity of taxable income. *Economic Journal, 127*, 297–329.

CHANG, Ming Chung. (2000). Rules and levels in the provision of public goods: The role of complementarities between the public good and the taxed commodities. *International Tax and Public Finance, 7*, 83–91.

CHRISTIANSEN, Vidar. (1981). Evaluation of public projects under optimal taxation. *Review of Economic Studies*, XLVIII, 447–457.

DAHLBY, B. (2008). *The marginal cost of public funds: Theory and applications*. MIT Press.

FRANK, R. H. (1999). *Luxury Fever: Why Money Fails to Satisfy in an Era of Excess*. Free Press.

FELDSTEIN, Martin. (1997). How big should government be? *National Tax Journal, 50*(2), 197–213.

JACOBS, B. (2018). The marginal cost of public funds is one at the optimal tax system. *Int Tax Public Finance, 25*, 883–912. https://doi.org/10.1007/s10797-017-9481-0

KAPLOW, Louis. (1996). The optimal supply of public goods and the distortionary cost of taxation. *National Tax Journal, 49*(4), 513–533.

KING, Mervyn A. (1986). A Pigovian rule for the optimum provision of public goods. *Journal of Public Economics, 30*, 273–291.

KONISHI, Hideo. (1995). A Pareto-improving commodity tax reform under a smooth nonlinear income tax. *Journal of Public Economics, 56*, 413–446.

MURPHY, Kevin M. & TOPEL, Robert. (2000). Medical research: What's it worth? *Milken Institute Review*, 1st Qtr, 23–30.

NG, Yew-Kwang (1987a). Relative-income effects and the appropriate level of public expenditure, *Oxford Economic Papers*, 293–300.

NG, Yew-Kwang. (1987b). Diamonds are a government's best friend: Burden-free taxes on goods valued for their values. *American Economic Review, 77*, 186–191.

NG, Yew-Kwang. (1993). Mixed diamond goods and anomalies in consumer theory: Upward-sloping compensated demand curves with unchanged diamondness. *Mathematical Social Sciences, 25*, 287–293.

NG, Yew-Kwang. (2000a). The optimal size of public spending and the distortionary cost of taxation. *National Tax Journal, 53*(2), 313–322.

NG, Yew-Kwang. (2000b). *Efficiency, Equality, and Public Policy: With a Case for Higher Public Spending*. Macmillan.

NG, Yew-Kwang. (2004). *Welfare Economics: Towards a More Complete Analysis*. Palgrave/Macmillan.

NG, Yew-Kwang & LIU, Po-Ting. (2003). Global environmental protection – solving the international public-good problem by empowering the United Nations through cooperation with WTO. *International Journal of Global Environmental Issues, 3*(4), 409–417.

OLDS, James & MILNER, Peter. (1954). Positive reinforcement produced by electrical stimulation of septal area and other regions of the rat brain. *Journal of Comparative Physiological Psychology, 47*, 419–427.

PIGOU, Arthur C. (1928). *Public Finance*. Macmillan.

STIGLITZ, Joseph J. (1988). *Economics of the Public Sector*. Norton.

WILSON, John D. (1991). Optimal public good provision with limited lump-sum taxation. *American Economic Review, 81*(1), 153–166.

Open Access This chapter is licensed under the terms of the Creative Commons Attribution 4.0 International License (http://creativecommons.org/licenses/by/4.0/), which permits use, sharing, adaptation, distribution and reproduction in any medium or format, as long as you give appropriate credit to the original author(s) and the source, provide a link to the Creative Commons license and indicate if changes were made.

The images or other third party material in this chapter are included in the chapter's Creative Commons license, unless indicated otherwise in a credit line to the material. If material is not included in the chapter's Creative Commons license and your intended use is not permitted by statutory regulation or exceeds the permitted use, you will need to obtain permission directly from the copyright holder.

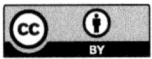

Chapter 16
Animal Welfare: Beyond Human Happiness

Abstract For animals capable of affective feelings (enjoyment and suffering), we should also be concerned with their welfare. Welfare biology studies at least three basic questions: Which (species are capable of welfare)? Whether (their welfare is positive)? How (to increase their welfare? As affective feelings entail energy costs, species not capable of making flexible choices are not capable of affective feelings. The fact that members of most species either starve to death or are eaten before successful mating, their net welfare is likely negative. We could decrease animal suffering by banning pointless cruelty and making the living conditions of our farmed animals better (like increasing cage sizes of chicken farming). However, the widespread reduction of extensive animal suffering including wild animals will largely have to be left after our significant scientific/technological, economic, and moral advances. Excessively strict guidelines on animal experimentation that inhibit scientific/technological advances may thus be counter-productive in animal salvation in the long run.

In our discussion of happiness, we have not covered two important issues:

1. On human happiness, we have not discussed the number of (human) individuals enjoying happiness or suffering negative happiness.
2. We also have not discussed happiness beyond humanity, particularly the issues of animal welfare/suffering.

The first problem is discussed in Appendix E. Here, we consider the second problem.

When we lived in Hong Kong over 1997, we shopped in the Shatin and Taipu wet markets often. We saw fish sellers cutting their life eels alive in halves, letting them wriggling in pain. I guess this is partly to attract attention and partly to show that their fish are very fresh. I argued with them, saying that the eels would be very painful. No one challenge me on this. But one seller replied, 'If I cannot sell my fish, I will also be painful.' It may be true that if only one seller cannot use this method while others could, he may sell less fish. However, if this cruel practice is prohibited by law, all fish sellers will still be able to sell their fish. Thus, such practices that inflict huge suffering on animals with no or negligible benefits to humans, should definitely be prohibited with strong sanctions against violators. I wrote on this and also emailed several relevant government offices in Hong Kong. Thus, I was happy to learn that the Hong Kong authority recently issued guidelines for the humane killing of fish for discussion. I hope that some good guidelines will soon be put into practice.

Though there is no such terrible cutting of life eels in halves in the West that I know of, the practice of wiping horses in racing is also something that should be banned. If all riders cannot wipe their horses, fair competition can still be carried on.

Why should we be concerned with animal welfare? As happiness is of intrinsic value and the rational ultimate objective (Chap. 5), the increase in our morality is ultimately reflected in our concern with the happiness of others. The degree of our morality is mainly measured by how much we are willing to sacrifice our own happiness to increase the happiness of others. The extent or scope of our morality is mainly defined by the set of these 'others' whom we are concerned with.

In ancient times, apart from oneself and family members, most people perhaps were mainly concerned with the bosses and the king/queen. After such movements like the glorious revolution in 1688, democracy gradually replaced imperial authority; the scope of moral concern increased to all nationals, and then to all human beings. This should increase further to all those with affective sentient feelings. This is likely to be a subset of all animal species. Ignoring the possible existence of gods, ghosts, and the like, there is no need to expand beyond this set, as plants and viruses are likely not affective sentients. Some biologists extend the concern to all living things inclusive of plants. This is excessive as life itself does not have intrinsic value. Thus, plants have only instrumental values by contributing to the happiness of animals with affective feelings.

Obviously, a Chinese individual will think that the morality of an English person who is only concerned with all individuals in England is lower than that of an English person who is not only concerned with all individuals in England, but also all individuals in the world, including the Chinese. Similarly, the morality of a person who is only concerned with all human individuals is lower than that of a person who is concerned not only with all human individuals, but also all animals with affective feelings. For an individual English/Chinese person, he may think that, with the same time and/or costs, it is more important to help one's country folks than foreigners. However, if we could help many persons in other countries with little costs, we should not preclude this option. Similarly, some persons may think that it is more important to be concerned with human welfare. However, if we could reduce animal suffering a lot at little costs on humans, we should also not preclude this option. Thus, we should not only be concerned with the welfare of other fellow human beings, but also with animal welfare.

Using the highest standard of morality, it may be argued that, all affective sentients, human or animal, should be equal; one welfare unit of any affective sentient, in itself (not ruling out the appropriate consideration of indirect effects on others and in the future) should have the same weight. While moral-philosophically valid, this highest level of morality is difficult to achieve in practice. However, we should at least have some degree of concern for animal welfare, avoiding unnecessarily inflicting suffering on animals at the very least.

Personally, I was very concerned with animal welfare long time ago. In 1995, I published a paper in an A* journal called *Biology and Philosophy*, proposing a field of study called 'welfare biology'. Two decades later, a scholar interested in animal welfare, Max Carpendale, interviewed me on the motivation and background of writing that paper. After seeing the interview on Carpendale's website, the editor of an academic journal, *Relations: Beyond Anthrocentrism,* published the interview in a 2015 issue of the journal (Carpendale 2015). In 2018, 80,000 hours also interviewed me on this and other issues. This paper on welfare biology seems to have attracted more attention than most of my papers in economics.

There are three basic questions in economics: What (to produce)? How? For whom? In my 1995 paper, I also raised three basic questions for welfare biology: Which (species are capable of welfare)? Whether (their welfare is positive or negative)? How (to increase their welfare)? Next, I used Darwinian theory of evolution and some basic economizing principle to help answer these basic questions, reaching some conclusions (but far from complete).

First, it may be argued that species without flexibility in their behavior have no affective feelings and hence are not capable of welfare or suffering. The generation of affective feelings requires energy costs. Thus, these feelings must contribute to the survival and reproduction fitness of the individual to avoid elimination from natural selection. However, the feelings of pleasure and pain themselves do not contribute to fitness. For example, when you see a tiger and feel terrified, this feeling alone does not help you to survive. This feeling must affect your activities, like running away or hide somewhere, to increase your chance for survival. Similarly, you feel nice seeing a beautiful lady; this nice feeling itself does not increase your fitness. It has to prompt you to mate with the lady to pass on your genes. If feelings of pleasure and pain do not increase your fitness but are costly, they will be selected against and hence cannot survive. They must affect your choices. For example, when seeing an animal, whether you should catch and eat it, or run away to prevent being eaten by it: the so-called 'fight or flight' decision is an important choice. The ability to make such flexible choices depending on the conditions of the situation (like the size of the animal, whether you have some weapon, etc.) which you may size up and decide on the spot, is important for your survival.

Some behavioral patterns of animals are completely fixed by genetic programs in advance. For example, a frog is born with the ability to jump around, swallowing small flying objects, as this help it to eat many insects and helps it to survive. However, if you put a frog in a confinement with many insects that do not fly, the frog will not be able to eat them and will starve to death. For another example, when we touch some very hot thing, our arm will withdraw itself to avoid being burnt. This reaction is automatic without thinking and is controlled by our spinal cord. If all the activities of a species consist only of such pre-programmed fixed patterns, it does not need to make flexible choices and hence it does not need affective feelings. Hence, natural selection will ensure that species not capable of any flexible choice will also not be capable of suffering and welfare. This helps us to answer the first basic question in welfare biology: Which species are capable of welfare? Only flexible species are. If we can establish that certain species completely lack flexibility, we may rule them out and not be concerned with causing any suffering on them. Though flexibility or not is still not easy to establish, the existence of affective feelings is even more subjective and difficult to establish. Hence, this first proposition in welfare biology is helpful.

Only flexible species are capable of welfare; however, this does not necessarily mean that we may rule out many species. The recently developed affective neuroscience shows that all mammals, and likely most if not all vertebrates, have affective feelings. In fact, 'hedonic brain mechanisms are largely shared between humans and other mammals' (Berridge and Kringelbach 2011, Abstract). Moreover, a paper in *Science* (Fossat et al. 2014) shows that even crayfish, which is not a vertebrate, has worries. When confined to a space with no escape, a crayfish secretes a chemical in its brain, a chemical we know that we will secrete in our brain only when we are worried. This strongly suggests, if not proves, that even crayfish is capable of worries. Also, arguably, worry is a higher form of unhappiness than just bodily pain. Thus, many species are capable of enjoyment and suffering.

The second basic question in welfare biology is: Whether the (net) welfare of animals are positive or negative? While not conclusive, my 1995 paper suggests that the answer is likely to be negative. This is based on the following two points. The first is based on the fact that, in most species, the number of offspring a mature female typically has over the lifespan is in hundreds, thousands, or more. In equilibrium and on average, only two of these many individual members will survive to adulthood and have successfully pass on their own offspring. The overwhelming majority of the others have a life of running away from predators in fear and finally got eaten or starve to death. Some of them may manage to survive until adulthood and be able to compete to mate. However, apart from the two lucky ones, the majority again fail to mate. It is difficult to imagine that a life like this will have more pleasures than pains. As there are many more unsuccessful than successful (in eventual mating and passing on the genes) individuals, overall negative welfare is likely. The second ground for this negative welfare conclusion is based on some economic-evolutionary theorizing. While my original 1995 paper suggests likely negative welfare from this ground, the issue is still being debated (Groff and Ng 2019).

According to happiness surveys, people in most countries are on average happy. We are also an animal species; how come our welfare is not negative? Happiness surveys are recent. If surveys were taken when we were still struggling on the life-and-death line, with most children starving to death or eaten by animals, our welfare would also likely be negative.

The third basic question in welfare biology is: How to increase animal welfare? Answers to this question could be very wide-ranging. However, to focus on some easy measures without too high costs, apart from banning pointless infliction of suffering on animals like the cutting of life eels in halves as mentioned above, an obvious area springing to mind is reducing suffering of animals we farm for food. We farm chicken, ducks, pigs, lambs, cows, etc. and eat their meat. If they suffer negative welfare in such a life, we are committing a double crime: make them suffer and then kill them for food.[1] On the other hand, if we could improve the living conditions of our farmed animals such as to increase their net welfare from negative to be positive, eating farmed animals is not morally bad. If we do not eat them, they would not have a chance of living at all. Then, there is no reason to be a vegetarian on moral grounds. The health ground for being a vegetarian or even a vegan is of dubious validity, as in our long history of evolution, we ate animals. The case for reducetarian (reducing instead of stopping eating animal products) is more supportable; see https://www.reducetarian.org/.

A simple way to reduce the suffering of our farmed animals is to increase their cage sizes, especially for the factory farming of chicken. The objection to this by producers that it would increase their costs and reduce their profits is based on incorrect economics. Chicken farming is largely under condition of free competition. Thus, in the long run, producers only earn normal profits. The institution of a drastic increase in cage sizes may lead initially to substantial increases in costs. However, in the long run, the increases in costs will be reflected in higher prices of chicken meat and eggs. The producers will still be earning normal profits. However, consumers will have to pay higher prices. Many of them would be glad to pay higher prices if the suffering of animals could be reduced substantially. For the majority of consumers who tend to over-consume meat, it is likely that higher prices will make them better off, just like a tax on cigarettes makes smokers better off (Gruber & Mullainathan 2005). For others, they still should pay higher prices, just like polluters should pay for the harm of pollution. (For animal suffering reduction, see also Ng 2016, 2019b.)

It may be thought that while the rich could pay for the higher prices easily, the poor will be harmed significantly. The issue of rich-poor or inequality is important but should be addressed separately. A person is rich or poor depending on her total purchasing power, not on the amount of chicken she consumes. Thus, we should pursue equality at the general equality policy focusing on total purchasing power. On specific measures including animal welfare or factory farming, we should follow the principle of efficiency supremacy. In this way, we can achieve the highest degree of equality at the same efficiency costs (Ng 2019a, Chap. 5).

For wild animals, we know even less. If my answer to the second basic question is correct, their net welfare is negative. However, it is more difficult to reduce their suffering (than that of our farmed animals). Some animal welfarists believe that we should at least not encroach upon their territories, reducing their living space. However, if their net welfare is negative, then while the contraction if their territories may involve transitory increases in suffering, in the long run, with lower number of individuals, their total suffering will also decrease. This is not clearly worse. In any case, I believe that, in the very long run, we have a duty to help increase the net welfare of even wild animals, hopefully to a positive level at least. Though not immediately feasible, we should try at least after significant advances economically, scientifically, technologically, and morally. Before this is feasible, we should try to prohibit pointless cruelty and reduce at least the suffering of our farmed animals as suggested above. Also, while we may have reasonable guidelines in experiments

---

[1] Not to mention the betrayal of the trust on us we create for animals; see Cooke (2019).

involving animals, we should not be too strict on this, as this would slow down scientific and technological advances upon which the salvation of animals will ultimately rely on.

References

BERRIDGE, Kent C. & KRINGELBACH, Morten L. (2011). Building a neuroscience of pleasure and well-being. *Theory, Research and Practice*, 1(3).

CARPENDALE, Max (2015). Welfare biology as an extension of biology: Interview with Yew-Kwang Ng, *Relations: Beyond Anthropocentrism*, 3(2): 197–202. Retrived from: http://www.ledonline.it/index.php/Relations/article/view/884

COOKE, S. (2019). Betraying animals. *Journal of Ethics, 23*, 183–200. https://doi.org/10.1007/s10892-019-09289-z

FOSSAT, Pascal, BACQUÉ-CAZENAVE, Julien, DE DEURWAERDÈRE, Philippe, DELBECQUE, Jean-Paul & CATTAERT, Daniel. (2014). Anxiety-like behavior in crayfish is controlled by serotonin. *Science, 344*(6189), 1293–1297.

GROFF, Z. & NG, Y-K. (2019). Does suffering dominate enjoyment in the animal kingdom? An update to welfare biology. *Biology & Philosophy, 34*, 40. https://doi.org/10.1007/s10539-019-9692-0

GRUBER, J., & MULLAINATHAN, S. (2005). Do cigarette taxes make smokers happier? *Advances in Economic Analysis & Policy, 5*, 1–43.

NG, Yew-Kwang (2016). How welfare biology and commonsense may help to reduce animal suffering, *Animal Sentience,* 2016.007. Target article for peer commentary. http://animalstudiesrepository.org/animsent/vol1/iss7/1/

NG, Yew-Kwang (2019a). *Markets and Morals: Justifying Kidney Sales and Legalizing Prostitution*, Cambridge University Press.

NG, Yew-Kwang (2019b). Human superiority is obvious but does not justify cruelty. *Animal Sentience* 23(36).

Open Access This chapter is licensed under the terms of the Creative Commons Attribution 4.0 International License (http://creativecommons.org/licenses/by/4.0/), which permits use, sharing, adaptation, distribution and reproduction in any medium or format, as long as you give appropriate credit to the original author(s) and the source, provide a link to the Creative Commons license and indicate if changes were made.

The images or other third party material in this chapter are included in the chapter's Creative Commons license, unless indicated otherwise in a credit line to the material. If material is not included in the chapter's Creative Commons license and your intended use is not permitted by statutory regulation or exceeds the permitted use, you will need to obtain permission directly from the copyright holder.

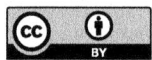

Appendix A
Resolving Some Moral Philosophical Controversies

By taking psychological happiness in the sense of feeling good instead of life satisfaction or 'attitudinal' happiness as of the ultimate value, many controversies in moral philosophy may be resolved. Just consider one example to illustrate the point here. Feldman (2004) advances an 'intrinsic attitudinal hedonism' theory of the good life. Due to taking the attitudinal happiness or rather life satisfaction as the focus, Feldman finds that the extrinsic satisfaction has to be excluded.

> When a person takes attitudinal pleasure in some state of affairs, he may take this pleasure in the state of affairs because he thinks it is related to some other state of affairs, and he takes pleasure in that other state of affairs. The most familiar instance of this sort of thing is the instrumental case. I take pleasure in the fact that the waiter is heading for our table. Why? Because I think he is bringing beer and peanuts, and I take pleasure in the fact that I soon will be enjoying them. … In cases like this, the person takes attitudinal pleasure in one state of affairs in virtue of the fact that he takes pleasure in others. In such cases, I say that the person is taking "extrinsic attitudinal pleasure.' (Feldman 2004, p. 63).

According to Feldman, only the intrinsic attitudinal pleasure of enjoying bear and peanuts is to be included, not the extrinsic one of anticipating the enjoyment. The intrinsic versus extrinsic distinction becomes irrelevant if we dispense with the 'attitudinal' requirement and go for happiness in the sense of feeling rather than life satisfaction. If the person also feels good when anticipating the enjoyment before actually eating, that pleasurable feeling is also a part of his subjective happiness. All actual positive feelings are to be counted positively and all negative feelings negatively, whether extrinsic or intrinsic in Feldman's sense.

Appendix B
Happiness as the Only Intrinsic Value: Further Opposing Arguments Considered

In commenting on happiness economics in general and on Layard (2005) in particular, Barrotta (2008, p.151) gives the example of the refusal of Freud to take drugs to reduce very painful conditions due to his desire to have clear thinking. If the reason to prefer clear thinking is to directly or indirectly contribute to his own and/or others' happiness in the future (perhaps through contribution to knowledge), there is no problem (no inconsistency with welfarism). If the clear thinking or autonomy does not contribute to happiness of anyone any time, the rationality of preferring it at the cost of much pain is questionable.

For another example, Benjamin et al. (2010, p. 3) find that 'predicted SWB [subjective well-being, similar to happiness] and choice coincide in our data 83 percent of the time'. Even for the rest, no conflict need be indicated as people could choose more income but say that the shorter hours option gives more happiness because the higher income could (or at least believed to) contribute to future happiness; the framing of their main question on p.6 does not rule out this likely possibility. Similarly, apparently non-utilitarian factors beyond happiness such as justice, rights, freedom, priority may all be justified on the important effects on others and the future.

Consider this conclusion: 'The evaluation of current mood is furthermore proposed to be situation-dependent such that in congruent situations (e.g. a celebration party) a positive mood leads to a positive evaluation of the positive mood and increased happiness, in incongruent situations (e.g. a funeral) a positive mood is evaluated negatively (Västfjäll and Gärling 2006) and thus paradoxically would lead to decreased happiness' (Gamble and Gärling 2011, 3rd page). Obviously, when one laughs on something funny at a funeral, it is not that one does not enjoy the funniness; rather, one is embarrassed by laughing at an inappropriate occasion. The reason for this is again considering the effects on others and in the future. One then refrains from laughing loudly in a funeral. This may reduce the positive enjoyment, and the embarrassment further reduces the net evaluation. However, the positive mood, to the extent it is felt, is still positive.

The point that negative feelings should count negatively in (net) happiness does not mean that pain or sufferings are useless. In fact, the pain sensation when say our fingers are burned triggers our withdrawal of our hand to avoid more damages and to teach us to avoid being burned in the future. However, the pain sensation as such is of negative value. It is also questionable to say that 'happiness and unhappiness are not ends, but means, and quite possibly "aspects of mechanisms that influence to act in the interests of our genes" (Nesse 2004, p. 1337)' (Nes 2010, p. 375). The problem of such statements is that they are based on confusing the (as-if) ends/means of our genes with our own ends/means. We are the feeling selves, not the unfeeling genes. It is quite true that our affective feelings were created/evolved to make us do things that help to spread our genes. However, the spreading of the unfeeling genes as such has no value. If the organisms that do have affective feelings have a lot more pain/unhappiness than happiness/pleasure and this miserable situation has no hope of being changed, the spreading of such genes is highly undesirable. Even for the reverse cases of more happiness, the valuable thing is the happy feelings, not the spreading of genes as such.

Consider the view 'that well-being is not so much an outcome or end state as it is a process of fulfilling or realizing one's daimon or true nature' (Deci & Ryan 2008, p. 2, describing the eudamonic view of well-being of that issue of *Journal of Happiness Studies*). If our true nature is interpreted as the biological one of survival and reproduction, a similar confusion of the (as-if) ends of our genes with our own ends may be involved. On the other hand, if our 'true nature' or eudaimonia are interpreted to require some elements of virtue (as required from Aristotle to Waterman), then the confusion is between happiness (that individuals and hence the society values ultimately) and morality, as discussed above. A morally very virtuous person may be very unhappy due to say sickness; a very happy person may be morally vicious by intentionally causing harm on others. While his happiness is valuable in itself, his causing of unhappiness on others may more than negate this. Again, once we take adequate account of the effects on others and the future, there is no need to go beyond the hedonic concept of happiness.

While many diverse desiderata (e.g. self-acceptance, self-determination, self-realization, relatedness, relationship, capability and functioning, environmental mastery, purpose) have been advanced by the believers in eudaimonia, let us consider here the need for autonomy emphasized by a number of authors. We may well have a natured and nurtured need for autonomy, as normally we will survive and thrive better with autonomy. Rationally, one may value autonomy only for its instrumental value in contributing directly (through fulfilling our desire to be autonomous) and indirectly (through its beneficial effects on other important things) towards our happiness. Thus, if I were mad and allowing me to be autonomous would cause great unhappiness upon myself and others much more than the small good feelings of being autonomous, I would not want to be autonomous.

For self-development, it could clearly be valuable now for its instrumental effects in contributing to the future happiness of oneself and possibly also of others. The fact that self-development is regarded as more important by younger people tends to support this interpretation. For the last dimension of contribution to others, it is also clear that if people find that happiness is the one that is valuable ultimately, then contribution to others must also be contributing to their happiness ultimately for it to be real contribution. Thus, provided happiness is taken to be net happiness counting

Appendix B: Happiness as the Only Intrinsic Value: Further Opposing Arguments ...

positive affective feelings positively and negative ones negatively, and provided the effects on others and in the future are not excluded, happiness needs only be of one dimension. Ultimately, it is the only thing that is really valuable.

Viewing happiness as the only ultimately valuable thing also does not conflict with the so-called 'hedonic paradox' that the intentional pursuit of happiness, especially if narrowly and excessively focused on the pleasures of the flesh, usually leads to unhappiness or less happiness (Veenhoven 2003; Martin 2008). To the extent that this is true, it means that a good way to achieve happiness is not to have myopic focus on the pleasures of the flesh in the short run, especially not excessively, but to do things more meaningful in contributing to one's own development and to the goodness (which has to be defined in terms of the effects on happiness ultimately) of the society in general. This does not negate the proposition that, ultimately speaking, only happiness is valuable.

Accepting happiness as the only ultimately valuable thing does not rule out the possibility that things other than happiness may be of interest for their instrumental values to happiness or for other purposes. For example, Waterman et al. (2008) and Huta and Ryan (2010) examine both 'hedonia' (similar to our concept of happiness here) and 'eudamonia' (which goes beyond happiness to require some elements of virtue) in affecting 'intrinsic motivation' or 'motives for acting'. Obviously, as both these factors do affect people's motives for acting, it is useful in studying the effects of both, even if one (like the present author) views virtue as ultimately being based on the contribution to happiness, especially to the happiness of others.

A specific implication of using the enjoyment/suffering sense of happiness (especially in contrast to using life satisfaction) may be briefly mentioned. It supports the Easterlin paradox (increases in incomes failing to increase happiness after a relatively low income level; Easterlin 1974, Easterlin et al. 2002) the validity of which has been questioned (Stevenson and Wolf 2008, 2013; Sacks et al. 2010; Angeles 2011). As reported in Graham (2011), Kahneman and Deaton (2010), in a study of 450,000 respondents in a Gallup daily survey of U.S. respondents from 2008 to 2009, found that hedonic wellbeing correlated less closely with income than did life satisfaction. Both 'correlated closely with income (in a log-linear manner) at the bottom end of the income ladder, but the correlation between hedonic well-being and income tapered off at about $75,000 per year'. (See Chap. 7 on further discussion of income and happiness.)

Regarding things other than welfare as intrinsically valuable is of questionable acceptability. For example, 'Non-economic modes of valuing typically result in intrinsic motivation. If one values an environmental good in itself or because of esthetic, historical or ecological reasons (valuation), one is likely to protect it regardless whether doing so helps to achieve some other goal (motivation)' (Neuteleers and Engelen 2015, p. 259). In my view, esthetic, historical and ecological values are valuable because they contribute to our welfare, not in themselves. If there is no sentients to appreciate them, they have no values.

On the other hand, it is also incorrect to say: 'If something has a price then it is not intrinsically valued' (Walsh 2015, p. 406). A pet animal has a price but also has intrinsic values as it has affective feelings. I have intrinsic value, at least to myself and my family members. However, I also have a price. I am willing to sell myself if possible, even for slavery, for say US $100 billion or higher. The extra money has no value to me myself, as my marginal utility/happiness of consumption is virtually zero. However, if I have a large sum of money like $100b., I think I could use it to do a lot of good, and this could increase a lot of welfare of other people and animals, such that even if I value the welfare of others and animals only at 1% of that of mine, it may still be worth it for me to slave for the rest of my life, provided that if I have at least 6 months to spend the money first. Arguably, I should be prepared to sell myself for something less than $100b; that is just a price I am willing to accept, not the minimum one.

In conclusion, despite the variety of objections to our central argument, I have never come across one that truly negates it. Most arguments ignore some relevant effects on others and in the future.

Appendix C
The Necessity of Cardinal Welfare for Rational Agents/Organisms

Using indifference/preference analysis, economists generally believe that as long as higher utility/welfare values are associated with higher preference levels, choices in accordance with the maximization of utility will be the same as choices maximizing preference, with different cardinal indices for the utility function. In this sense, utility needs only be ordinal. Does this mean that utility/welfare values need not be cardinal for the maximization of utility/welfare to be consistent with fitness maximization, even though fitness itself is cardinal? This appendix shows that, at least when choices involving risk are involved, as almost always true in the real world of uncertainty, welfare values for rational agents have to be cardinal and similar to fitness values in their cardinality for rational choices to be consistent with expected fitness maximization.

For simplicity, let us be content with the illustration of the central point that can be seen to be applicable more generally. Consider that a rational organism (as happiness studies are currently virtually exclusively concerned with Homo sapiens, this rationality assumption is certainly valid) is faced with the choice between two actions a and b, with two possible states of nature x and y with equal probability of 50% each (again purely for simplicity without real loss of generality). Let $F(j, k)$ and $W(j, k)$ be the fitness and welfare values of actions $j = a, b$ and states of nature $k = x, y$ respectively. Consider a specific case, without real loss of generality (since it is obvious that the point made with the specific numbers here also applies more generally) where.

(1) $F(b, y) = 22 > F(a, y) = 20 > F(a, x) = 10 > F(b, x) = 5$.

The maximization of expected fitness requires the choice of action a. If $W(j, k)$ is equal to $F(j, k)$ for all values of j, k, the required expected fitness maximization choice will coincide with that of the maximization of expected welfare values. As F is cardinal, so is W. However, if $W(j, k)$ is made only having the same ordinal ranking but not the same cardinal values as $F(j, k)$, in general, the maximization of expected welfare values by rational agents/organisms (required to satisfy compelling rationality axioms; see Ng 1984) does not in general coincide with that of expected fitness maximization. For example if we have.

(2) $W(b,y) = 50 > W(a,y) = 20 > W(a,x) = 10 > W(b,x) = 5$,

the ordering of the various welfare values for all the four outcomes under consideration is exactly the same as that of the fitness values in (1) above. However, expected welfare maximization in this case dictates the choice of action b, contrary to the requirement of expected fitness maximization.

Obviously, in order that the maximization of expected welfare always dictates the same action as that for expected fitness maximization, the welfare values under different outcomes have either to be the same as the fitness values or are some linear transformation of the latter, i.e. have to be not only having the same ranking, but also having the same cardinal numbers unique up to a linear transformation. This makes welfare values cardinal but not yet in a ratio scale. For the latter (full cardinality), we need to pin point the point of zero welfare. This is the point when an organism (individual) feels neither pleasure nor pain. For most people, this is the case when the individual is not doing anything enhancing or detrimental to fitness, directly or indirectly through expectation. Why is a zero welfare value associated with zero implication for fitness? This is so because it is costly (energy consumption) to produce either pleasure or pain. Thus, activities with no implication for fitness should neither be penalized nor rewarded. (For more details, see Ng 1995.)

Appendix D
A Problem in Happiness Measurement

This problem arises when only a fixed scale (e.g. from 0 to 10, or from 0 to 100) is allowed for the range of happiness reported. Suppose that I am currently very happy and report my happiness level as being 90 out of 100. Suppose my net happiness amount were to double (not to mention a three or fourfold increase) some years from now (when I already report an index of 90). Using the scale of 0–100, I cannot report my happiness as 180. I would probably report 95. However, this problem is due to the confinement to the range 0–100. When people are confined to a scale of 0–10 or 0–100, people tend to use the scale somewhat between the normal numerical scale and something like either the logarithmic or the Richter scale (used to measure earthquakes; an increase by one signifies a tenfold increase). While different persons may use the scale to represent different levels of happiness, personally I am inclined to use a scale like the one in Fig. D.1, where the horizontal axis is the scale between 0–100 and the vertical axis is my cardinal amount of happiness over a certain period. Such a scale allows the coverage of a larger range of variation of happiness amount and also allows more significant differences over the non-extreme range. If one were to use a normal numerical scale, it will appear as a straight line in Fig. D.1. Then there are an upper and a lower bounds for happiness level beyond which one has to use the same number 100 (for upper) or zero (for lower) even for further variations.

Strictly speaking, the non-linearity in the happiness scale makes the averaging, summation, and multiplication of happiness indices (with life expectancy in particular) of questionable validity. This difficulty can be overcome if a linear scale is used as could be obtained by using the method of happiness measurement based on the number of just perceivable increments as discussed in Chap. 6. Before such more reliable measures of happiness are used, existing measures may yet be used as the best we have available. Moreover, the use of happiness measures unadjusted for the non-linearity (see Fig. D.1 and the associated discussion above) may yet serves as a desirable adjustment for those (e.g. Veenhoven and Kalmijn 2005 who propose the measure of 'inequality-adjusted happiness') who wish to take into account of the

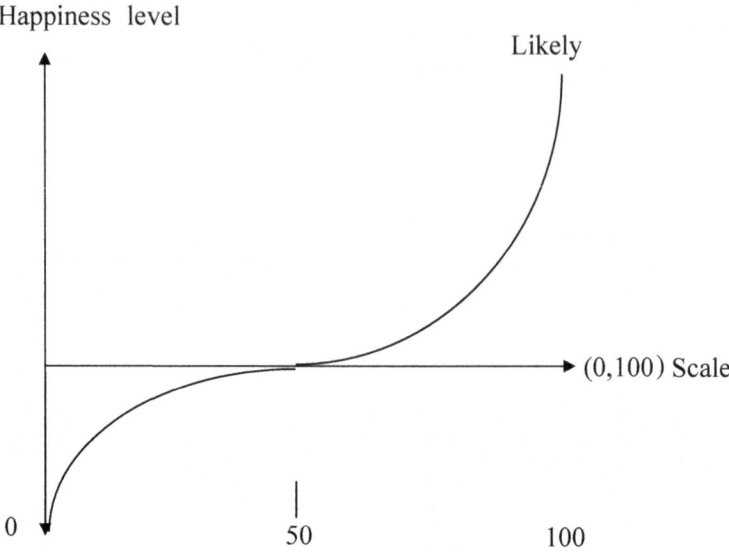

Fig. D.1 Reported happiness levels may be non-linear

equality in the distribution of happiness level.[1] Most happiness indices obtained in actual surveys fall between 40 and 80 (for a scale of 0–100). Egalitarian adjustments require counting the same increments of happiness indices at the high end (70–90) as less important than those at the low end (40–60). As may be seen from Fig. D.1, the needed adjustment to account for the likely non-linearity requires exactly the reverse adjustment. Of course, the two opposite adjustments may not be exactly offsetting to each other. However, they may be roughly or at least partly offsetting.

---

[1] Personally, I do not believe in the relevance of equality in the ultimate objective. Inequality in income is undesirable both because of the diminishing marginal utility/welfare of income and because of the indirect undesirable effects of inequality in reducing happiness through for example reducing social cohesion. Since happiness is already the ultimate objective, we can neither have diminishing marginal happiness of happiness nor further indirect effects, except in an intertemporal framework where the happiness in the future has not yet been accounted for. Either accounting for this intertemporal effect or ignoring it, an objective function that is not linear in individual happiness can be shown to violate some compelling axiom, i.e. treating a perceivable increment of happiness as less important than a not perceivable one; see Ng (1975, 1984). Moreover, the argument for the utilitarian social welfare function (Ng 2000b, Chap. 5) supports not taking into account inequality in the ultimate objective. (These are briefly discussed in Sect. 3.) Also, Ott (2005) shows that higher average happiness tends to go with higher equality in happiness.

Appendix E
A Solution of the Moral Philosophical Problem of Optimal Population Size

In the main text, we have not considered issues when the population size or the number of individuals is a variable. When population size may change, the most prominent issue is: What is the relevant social welfare that should be maximized when the set or just the number of individuals (to simplify the issue) is a variable. Here, we have the centuries-old issue of average versus total welfare maximization in moral philosophy. Should we prefer a society (or an alternative for the society) with higher average (i.e. per-person) welfare, or one with higher total welfare (= average welfare times the number of individuals concerned). Classical utilitarianism goes for the maximization of total welfare. The problem of this is that it leads to the so-called Repugnant Conclusion. As long as the number of individuals is increased sufficiently to offset the decrease in average welfare, we have to prefer an alternative with an average life barely worth living (with positive welfare but arbitrarily close to zero).

The apparent dismal result of the Repugnant Conclusion leads many to go for average welfare maximization. However, this option has a worse implication; it violates the compelling Mere Addition Principle: The addition of additional happy individuals (i.e. with positive net welfare levels) without decreasing the welfare level of any existing person should be regarded as a good change. Obviously, if the average welfare level of the additional individuals is lower than that of the existing individuals, the larger population size leads to lower average welfare level, though the level of total welfare may increase enormously. If we have to choose two alternatives (with relevant ultimate outcomes all included; no relevant effects on the future left unaccounted for) of: A. 1000 units of net welfare for 10 individuals only; B. 1100 units of net welfare for these same 10 individuals, plus 990 units for an additional million individuals, we have to prefer A, denying the additional one million individuals to enjoy happy lives, even at a bonus of making the pre-existing 10 individuals also happier, as the average welfare level is lower in B than in A. Clearly, this is bad moral philosophy.

The above dilemma between average and total welfare maximization has troubled the moral philosophy circles for centuries with no generally acceptable 'solution'. Some position between average and total welfare is also not an acceptable solution as it just means both the violation of the Mere Addition Principle to some extent and having the Repugnant Conclusion in some degree. This population size dilemma was perceptively discussed by Parfit (1984) in his very readable monograph. Parfit believes that a Theory X that avoids the Repugnant Conclusion and satisfies the Mere Addition Principle as well as some other compelling conditions exists but he could not find it. However, after reading Parfit's beautiful discussion, I show that Theory X does not exist (Ng 1989). Any theory/principle that meets the Mere Addition Principle and some compelling conditions (including Non-antiegalitarianism: A more equally distributed welfare profile with no lower level of total welfare cannot be worse) cannot avoid the Repugnant Conclusion. While this seems a devastating result in the moral philosophy of population size, I also argue that the so-called Repugnant Conclusion is not really repugnant (For support from 29 authors, see Zuber, et.al. 2021.). As well, I offer a way out. At the level of pure moral philosophy, especially when we are comparing two alternative ultimate outcomes unrelated to our own interest, we should morally use the principle of total welfare maximization, meeting the Mere Addition Principle and other compelling conditions. However, for choices that may affect our own welfare, we may not be prepared to sacrifice our own welfare significantly, even if this could lead to much larger increase in welfare of potential people (people not yet born but could be born under some relevant alternatives). Similarly, a rich person may agree that donating a high proportion of his wealth will increase social welfare, but may only donate a very small proportion. This is a question of ideal morality versus self-interest. (The rich person case may also involve the publicness aspect; if all rich persons donate, he may be glad to do so.) This is my resolution of the optimal population dilemma in moral philosophy that I discuss in some details in my 1989 paper.

References

ANGELES, Luis. (2011). A closer look at the Easterlin paradox. *Journal of Socio-Economics,40*, 67–73.
ARISTOTLE. (1985). Nicomachean Ethics. In: T. Irwin (Trans). Hackett, Indianapolis.
BARROTTA, P. (2008). Why economists should be unhappy with the economics of happiness. *Economics and Philosophy,24*(2), 145–165.
BENJAMIN, Daniel J., HEFFETZ, Ori, KIMBALL, Miles S. & REES-JONES, Alex (2010). Do people seek to maximize happiness? evidence from new surveys, Working Paper 16489, *National Bureau of Economic Research*. Retrieved from: http://www.nber.org/papers/w16489
DECI, Edward L. & RYAN, Richard M. (2008). Hedonia, eudaimonia, and well-being: An introduction. *Journal of Happiness Studies,9*, 1–11.
EASTERLIN, Richard A., ed. (2002) . *Happiness in Economics*.Elgar Reference Collection.International Library of Critical Writings in Economics, vol. 142. Cheltenham, U.K. and Northampton, Mass.: Elgar; distributed by American International Distribution Corporation, Williston, VT.
FELDMAN, Fred. (2004). *Pleasure and the Good Life*. Oxford University Press.
GAMBLE, Amelie & GÄRLING, Tommy. (2011). The relationships between life satisfaction, happiness, and current mood. *Journal of Happiness Studies,3*(1), 31–45.
GRAHAM, Carol (2011) Happiness measures as a guide to development policy? Promise and potential pitfalls. Paper presented at the Annual Meetings of the American Economic Association, Denver, January 7.
HUTA, Veronika & RYAN, Richard M. (2010). Pursuing pleasure or virtue: The differential and overlapping well-being benefits of hedonic and eudaimonic motives. *Journal of Happiness Studies,11*, 735–762.
KAHNEMAN, Daniel & DEATON, Angus. (2010). *Does money buy happiness…or just a better life*. Princeton University.
LAYARD, Richard. (2005). *Happiness: Lessons from a New Science*. Penguin.
MARTIN, Mike W. (2008). Paradoxes of happiness. *Journal of Happiness Studies,9*, 171–184.
NES, Ragnhild Bang. (2010). Happiness in behaviour genetics: Findings and implications. *Journal of Happiness Studies,11*(3), 369–381.
NESSE, Randolph. (2004). Natural selection and the elusiveness of happiness. *Philosophical Transactions of the Royal Society of London, Series B,359*, 1333–1347.
NEUTELEERS, S. & ENGELEN, B. (2015). Talking money: How market-based valuation can undermine environmental protection. *Ecological Economics,117*, 253–260.
NG, Yew-Kwang (1975). Bentham or Bergson? Finite sensibility, utility functions, and
NG, Yew-Kwang. (1984). Expected subjective utility: Is the Neumann-Morgenstern utility the same as the neoclassical's? *Social Choice and Welfare,1*(3), 177–186.

NG, Yew-Kwang. (1989). What should we do about future generations? The impossibility of Parfit's theory X. *Economics and Philosophy,5*(2), 235–253.

NG, Yew-Kwang (1995). Towards welfare biology: Evolutionary economics of animal consciousness and suffering. *Biology and Philosophy*, 10(3): 255–285. Retrieved from: http://www.springerlink.com/content/uj81758r18717777/

NG, Yew-Kwang. (2000). *Efficiency, Equality, and Public Policy: With a Case for Higher Public Spending.* Macmillan.

OTT, Jan. (2005). Level and inequality of happiness in nations: Does greater happiness of a greater number imply greater inequality in happiness? *Journal of Happiness Studies,6*(4), 397–420.

PARFIT, Derek. (1984). *Reasons and Persons.* Clarendon Press.

SACKS, Daniel W., STEVENSON, Betsey & WOLFERS, Justin (2010). Subjective well-being, income, economic development and growth, CESifo Working Paper No. 3206. Retrieved from: http://www.ifo.de/portal/pls/portal/docs/1/1185210.PDF.

STEVENSON, Betsey & WOLFERS, Justin (2008). Economic growth and subjective well-being: Reassessing the Easterlin Paradox. *Brookings Papers on Economic Activity*, Spring.

STEVENSON, Betsey & WOLFERS, Justin. (2013). Subjective well-being and income: Is there any evidence of satiation? *American Economic Review Papers and Proceedings,103*(3), 598–604.

VÄSTFJÄLL, Daniel & GÄRLING, Tommy. (2006). Preferences for negative emotions. *Emotion,6*, 326–329.

VEENHOVEN, Ruut. (2003). Hedonism and happiness. *Journal of Happiness Studies,4*(4), 437–457.

WALSH, A. (2015). Compensation for blood plasma donation as a distinctive ethical hazard: Reformulating the commodification objection. *HEC Forum, 27(4)* (pp. 401–416). Springer.

WATERMAN, Alan S., SCHWARTZ, Seth J. & CONTI, Regina. (2008). The implications of two conceptions of happiness (hedonic enjoyment and eudaimonia) for the understanding of intrinsic motivation. *Journal of Happiness Studies,9*, 41–79.

VEENHOVEN, Ruut & KALMIJN, Wim. (2005). Inequality-adjusted happiness in nations: Egalitarianism and utilitarianism married in a new index of societal performance. *Journal of Happiness Studies,6*, 421–455.

ZUBER, Stéphanie, et al. (2021). What should we agree on about the repugnant conclusion? *Utilitas*, 1–5, doi:https://doi.org/10.1017/S095382082100011X.

Uncited References

AHUVIA, Aaron C. & FRIEDMAN, Douglas C. (1998). Income, consumption, and subjective well-being: Toward a composite macromarketing model. *Journal of Macromarketing,18*(2), 153–168.

ANTONOVSKY, Anna. (1996). The salutogenic model as a theory to guide health promotion. *Health Promotion International,11*(1), 11–18.

BLACKSON, Thomas. (2009). On Feldman's theory of happiness. *Utilitas,21*(3), 393–400.

BLANCHFLOWER, David G. & OSWALD, Andrew J. (2004). Money, sex and happiness: An empirical study. *The Scandinavian Journal of Economics,106*(3), 393–415.

BRICKMAN, Phillip, COATES, Dan and JANOFF-BULMAN, Ronnie. (1978). Lottery winners and accident victims: Is happiness relative? *Journal of Personality and Social Psychology,36*, 917–927.

CLARK, A. E. & OSWALD, A. J. (1996). *Satisfaction and comparison income, Discussion paper 419.* Essex University.

CLARK, Andrew E., et al. (2014). What predicts a successful life? A life-course model of well-being. Economic Journal, forthcoming.

DI TELLA, Rafael & MACCULLOCH, Robert (2000). Partisan social happiness, paper presented at the Economics and Happiness Conference, Nuffield College, Oxford, 11–12 (Feb).

DJANKOV, S., LA PORTA, R., LOPEZ-DE-SILANES, F. & SHLEIFER, A. (2002). The regulation of entry. *The Quarterly Journal of Economics,117*(1), 1–37. https://doi.org/10.1162/003355302 753399436

DOCES, J. A. & WOLAVER, A. (2019). Are We *All* Predictably Irrational? An Experimental Analysis. *Political Behavior*. DOI: https://doi.org/10.1007/s11109-019-09579-0

EASTERLIN, Richard A., MORGAN, R., SWITEK, M, WANG, Fei. (2012). China's life satisfaction, 1990–2010. *PNAS,109*, 9775–9780.

EASTERLIN, Richard A., WANG, Fei and WANG, Shun. (2017). Growth and happiness in China, 1990–2015. *World Happiness Report,2017*, 48.

FONTAINE, P. (2018) Altruism, history of the concept. In: Macmillan Publishers Ltd (eds) *The New Palgrave Dictionary of Economics*. Palgrave Macmillan, London

FRIJTERS, P. & BEATTON, T. (2012). The mystery of the U-shaped relationship between happiness and age. *Journal of Economic Behavior & Organization,82*(2–3), 525–542. https://doi.org/10.1016/j.jebo.2012.03.008

FRIJTERS, Paul (1999), 'Do individuals try to maximize general satisfaction?', typescript

FURNHAM, Adrian & CHENG, Helen. (1999). Personality as predictor of mental health and happiness in the East and West. *Personality and Individual Differences,27*, 395–403.

GIUBILINI, A., CAVIOLA, L., MASLEN, H., et al. (2019). Nudging Immunity: The Case for Vaccinating Children in School and Day Care by Default. *HEC Forum,31*, 325–344. https://doi.org/10.1007/s10730-019-09383-7

GRAHAM, Carol (2012). *Happiness Around the World: The Paradox of Happy Peasants and Miserable Millionaires*. Oxford University Press.

GRAHAM, Carol (2017). *Happiness for All? Unequal Hopes and Lives in Pursuit of hthe American Dream*. Princeton University Press.

HANDS, D.W. (2020). Libertarian paternalism: Taking Econs seriously. *International Review of Economics*. https://doi.org/10.1007/s12232-020-00349-7

HEADLEY, Bruce and WEARING, Alexander (1991). Subjective well-being: a stocks and flows framework. In Argyle, M. and Schwarz, N. (eds.). *Subjective Well-Being*. Oxford: Pergamon.

HELLIWELL, John F. & AKNIN, Lara B. (2018). Expanding the social science of happiness. *Nature Human Behaviour,2018*, 1.

HELLIWELL, John F., BARRINGTON-LEIGH, Chris, HARRIS, Anthony & HUANG Haifang (2010). International evidence on the social context of well-being, In Diener et al. (Eds.), *International differences in well-being* (pp. 291–327).

HELLIWELL, John F., HUANG, Haifang & WANG, Shun. (2017). The social foundations of world happiness. *World Happiness Report,2017*, 8.

HINDRIKS, Frank, and DOUVEN, Igor. (2018). Nozick's experience machine: An empirical study. *Philosophical Psychology,31*(2), 278–298.

JOHNSTONE, Brick, , et al. (2017). Selflessness as a universal neuropsychological foundation of spiritual transcendence: Validation with Christian, Hindu, and Muslim traditions. *Mental Health, Religion & Culture,20*(2), 175–187.

KAHNEMAN, D. & TVERSKY, A. (1996). On the reality of cognitive illusions: A reply to Gigerenzer's critique. *Psychological Review,103*(3), 582–591. https://doi.org/10.1037/0033-295X.103.3.582

KAHNEMAN, Daniel (2000). Experienced utility and objective happiness: A moment-based approach. In D. Kahneman and A. Tversky (Eds), *Choices, Values and Frames*. New York, NY, US: Russell Sage Foundation, Cambridge University Press.

KENNY, Charles. (1999). Does growth cause happiness, or does happiness cause growth? *Kyklos,52*, 3–26.

KNIGHT, John & GUNATILAKA, Ramani. (2010). The rural-urban divide in China: Income but not happiness? *Journal of Development Studies,46*(3), 506–534.

KUBOVY, M., KAHNEMAN, D., DIENER, E. & SCHWARZ, N. (1999). *Well-being: The foundations of hedonic psychology*.

LACEY, Heather P., SMITH, Dylan M. & UBEL, Peter A. (2006). Hope I die before I get old: Mispredicting happiness across the adult lifespan. *Journal of Happiness Studies,7*(2), 167–182.
LAMPE, Kurt (2015). *The Birth of Hedonism: The Cyrenaic Philosophers and Pleasure as a Way of Life.* Princeton University Press.
LANE, Robert E. (2000). *The Loss of Happiness in Market Democracies.* Yale University Press.
LARSEN, Randy J. & FREDRICKSON, Barbara L. (1999). Measurement issues in emotion research, Chapter 3 In D. Kahneman, E. Diener & N. Schwarz, *Well-Being: Foundations of Hedonic Psychology* (pp. 40–60).
LAVALLEE, Loraine F., HATCH, P. M., MICHALOS, Alex C. & MCKINLEY, Tara. (2007). Development of the contentment with life assessment scale (clas): Using daily life experiences to verify levels of self-reported life satisfaction. *Social Indicators Research,83*, 201–244.
LIANG, H., CHEN, C., LI, F., et al. (2020). Mediating effects of peace of mind and rumination on the relationship between gratitude and depression among Chinese university students. *Current Psychology,39*, 1430–1437. https://doi.org/10.1007/s12144-018-9847-1
LOEWENSTEIN, George and SHANE Frederick (1998). Hedonic adaptation: From the bright side to the dark side. In KAHNEMAN, Daniel, DIENER, Ed, and SCHWARTZ, Norbert (ed.) *Understanding Well-Being: Scientific Perspectives on Enjoyment and Suffering*, New York: Russell Sage.
LOH, Jonathan & WACKERNAGEL, Mathis (Eds.) (2004). *Living Planet Report 2004.* Switzerland: Gland.
LYUBOMIRSKY, S., KING, L. & DIENER, E. (2005). The benefits of frequent positive affect: Does happiness lead to success? *Psychological Bulletin,131*, 803–855.
MAN, X. & CAO, H. (2020). Prevalence and protective factors of psychological distress among left-behind children in rural China: A study based on national data. *Journal of Child and Family Studies,29*, 1274–1283. https://doi.org/10.1007/s10826-020-01703-7
MASLOW, A. H. (1954). *Motivation and personality.* Harper and Row.
MASLOW, Abraham H. & LOWRY, Richard J. (1973). *Dominance, Self-Esteem, Self-Actualization: Germinal Papers of A. H. Maslow*, California: Brooks/Cole Pub. Co.
MCCARTHY, N. (2018). Air Pollution Contributed To More Than 6 Million Deaths In 2016. Forbes, Apr 18, 2018.
NG, Siang and NG, Yew-Kwang (forthcoming). Welfare-reducing growth despite individual and government optimization, *Social Choice and Welfare*.
NG, Yew-Kwang & HO, Lok Sang (2006). Happiness and Public Policy: An Introduction. In *Happiness and Public Policy: Theory, Case Studies, and Implications.* London: Palgrave/Macmillan.
NG, Yew-Kwang. (1990). Welfarism and utilitarianism: A rehabilitation. *Utilitas,2*(2), 171–193.
NG, Yew-Kwang. (1999). Utility, informed preference, or happiness? *Social Choice and Welfare,16*(2), 197–216.
NG, Yew-Kwang (2000a). From Preference to Happiness: Towards a more Complete Welfare Economics, Keynote paper, International Conference on 'Economics and the Pursuit of Happiness', Nuffield College, Oxford, February 2000.
NG, Yew-Kwang (2000b). Why do economists overestimate the costs of public spending? *Newsletter of the Royal Economic Society, U.K.*, Issue 110, July, 5–7.
NG, Yew-Kwang (2001). Is public spending good for you?, *World Economics,* invited but refereed contribution, April-June 2001, 2(2): 1–17.
NG, Yew-Kwang (2002). The East-Asian happiness gap, *Pacific Economic Review,* 2002, 7(1): 51–63.
NG, Yew-Kwang. (2008). Happiness studies: Ways to improve comparability and some public policy implications. *Economic Record,84*, 253–266.
NG, Yew-Kwang (2018). Ten rules for public economic policy, *Economic Analysis and Policy*, forthcoming.
OSHIO, Takashi & URAKAWA, Kunio. (2014). The association between perceived income inequality and subjective well-being: Evidence from a social survey in Japan. *Social Indicators Research,116*, 755–770.

OSWALD, A. J., PROTO, E. & SGROI, D. (2015). Happiness and productivity. *Journal of Labor Economics,33*(4), 789–822.
OSWALD, Andrew J. & WU, Stephen. (2010). Objective confirmation of subjective measures of human well-being: Evidence from the USA. *Science,327*(5965), 576–579.
PINQUART, Martin. (2001). Age differences in perceived positive affect, negative affect, and affect balance in middle and old age. *Journal of Happiness Studies,2*, 375–405.
RAM, Rati. (2009). Government spending and happiness of the population: Additional evidence from large cross-country samples. *Public Choice,138*, 483–490. https://doi.org/10.1007/s11127-008-9372-0
RYAN, Richard M., CHIRKOV, Valery I., LITTLE, Todd D., SHELDON, Kennon M., TIMOSHINA, Elena & DECI, Edward L. (1999). The American dream in Russia: Extrinsic aspirations and well-being in two cultures. *Personality and Social Psychology Bulletin,25*(12), 1509–1524.
STONE, Arthur A., SHIFFMAN, Saul S. & DeVRIES, Marten W. (1999).Ecological momentary assessment, Chapter 2 in D. Kahneman, E. Diener& N. Schwarz. *Well-being: The foundations of hedonic psychology* (pp. 26–39). New York, NY, US: Russell Sage Foundation.
TACHIBANAKI, Toshiaki (Ed.) (2016). *Advances in Happiness Research: A Comparative Perspective*, Springer.
TERRADAILY (2005). Terradaily: News about Planet Earth, Retrieved from: http://www.terradaily.com/reports/China_Warns_Of_FiveFold_Increase_In_Air_Pollution_In_15_Years.html.
TERRADAILY (2006), Terradaily: News about planet earth, Retrieved from: http://www.terradaily.com/reports/400_000_People_In_China_Die_Prematurely_From_Air_Pollution_Annually_Expert.html.
TREMBLAY, Leon and SCHULTZ, Wolfram. (1999). Relative reward preference in primate orbitofrontal cortex. *Nature,398*, 704–708.
UNANOE, Wenceslao (2017). Subjective wellbeing measures to inform public policies, In *Happiness Transforming the Development Landscape* (pp. 60–79). The Centre for Bhutan Studies and GNH.
United Nations' Department of Economic and Social Affairs (2008), *Millennium Development Goals Indicators*. Retrieved from: https://unstats.un.org/unsd/mdg/Host.aspx?Content=Indicators%2fOfficialList.htm
VEENHOVEN, Ruut. (2002). Why social policy needs subjective indicators. *Social Indicators Research,58*(1–3), 33–45.
VEENHOVEN, Ruut (2017). Measures of Happiness: Which to Choose? *Metrics of Subjective Well-Being: Limits and Improvements*. Springer, Cham, 2017.65–84.
VENTEGODT, Søren. (1996). *Measuring the Quality of Life: From Theory to Practice*. Forskningscentrets Forlag.
VIALE, R. (2019). Architecture of the mind and libertarian paternalism: Is the reversibility of system 1 nudges likely to happen? *Mind & Society,18*, 143–166. https://doi.org/10.1007/s11299-019-00218-z
VISHKIN, A., BLOOM, P. B. N. & TAMIR, M. (2019). Always look on the bright side of life: Religiosity, emotion regulation and well-being in a Jewish and Christian sample. *Journal of Happiness Studies,20*(2), 427–447.
WALSH, David and GILLESPIE, Austin. (1990). *Designer Kids: Consumerism and Competition: When is it all too much?* Deaconess Press.
WALTON, Michael (1997). The maturation of the East Asian miracle. *Finance & Development,* Sept.
WATANABE, Masataka. (1999). Neurobiology: Attraction is relative not absolute. *Nature,398*, 661–663.
YE, Dezhu, NG, Yew-Kwang, LIAN, Yujun. (2015). Culture and Happiness. *Social Indicators Research,123*(2), 519–547.
ZHOU, Haiou. (2012). A new framework of happiness survey and evaluation of national wellbeing. *Social Indicators Research,108*(3), 491–507.

Printed by Printforce, United Kingdom